Computer-Aided
Drug Design

Computer-Aided
Drug Design

Anees Ahmad Siddiqui MPharm, PhD
Department of Pharmaceutical Chemistry
School of Pharmaceutical Education and Research
Jamia Hamdard, New Delhi 110062

Harish Kumar MPharm, PhD
Department of Pharmaceutical Sciences
PDM University, Haryana

Subuhi Khisal MPharm
Department of Pharmaceutical Chemistry
School of Pharmaceutical Education and Research
Jamia Hamdard, New Delhi 110062

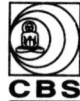

CBS

CBS Publishers & Distributors Pvt Ltd

New Delhi • Bengaluru • Chennai • Kochi • Kolkata • Mumbai
Bhopal • Bhubaneswar • Hyderabad • Jharkhand • Nagpur • Patna • Pune • Uttarakhand • Dhaka (Bangladesh)

Computer-Aided
Drug Design

ISBN: 978-93-87964-35-8

Copyright © Authors and Publisher

First Edition: 2020

Published by Satish Kumar Jain and produced by Varun Jain for

CBS Publishers & Distributors Pvt Ltd
4819/XI Prahlad Street, 24 Ansari Road, Daryaganj, New Delhi 110 002, India.
Ph: 23289259, 23266861, 23266867   Fax: 011-23243014   Website: www.cbspd.com
e-mail: delhi@cbspd.com; cbspubs@airtelmail.in.
Corporate Office: 204 FIE, Industrial Area, Patparganj, Delhi 110 092
Ph: 4934 4934   Fax: 4934 4935   e-mail: publishing@cbspd.com; publicity@cbspd.com

Branches

* **Bengaluru:** Seema House 2975, 17th Cross, K.R. Road,
  Banasankari 2nd Stage, Bengaluru 560 070, Karnataka
  Ph: +91-80-26771678/79   Fax: +91-80-26771680   e-mail: bangalore@cbspd.com
* **Chennai:** 7, Subbaraya Street, Shenoy Nagar, Chennai 600 030, Tamil Nadu
  Ph: +91-44-26680620, 26681266   Fax: +91-44-42032115   e-mail: chennai@cbspd.com
* **Kochi:** 42/1325, 1326, Power House Road, Opposite KSEB Power House,
  Ernakulam 682 018, Kochi, Kerala
  Ph: +91-484-4059061-65   Fax: +91-484-4059065   e-mail: kochi@cbspd.com
* **Kolkata:** 6/B, Ground Floor, Rameswar Shaw Road, Kolkata 700 014, West Bengal
  Ph: +91-33-22891126, 22891127, 22891128   e-mail: kolkata@cbspd.com
* **Mumbai:** 83-C, Dr E Moses Road, Worli, Mumbai 400018, Maharashtra
  Ph: +91-22-24902340/41   Fax: +91-22-24902342   e-mail: mumbai@cbspd.com

Representatives

* **Bhopal** 0-8319310552 • **Bhubaneswar** 0-9911037372 • **Hyderabad** 0-9885175004 • **Jharkhand** 0-9811541605
* **Nagpur** 0-9421945513 • **Patna** 0-9334159340 • **Pune** 0-9623451994 • **Uttarakhand** 0-9716462459
* **Dhaka (Bangladesh)** 01912-003485

Printed at Glorius Printers, Daryaganj, Delhi, India

Preface

The Pharmacy Council of India implemented the new syllabus for BPharm course throughout India in 2017. The syllabus comprises a new subject namely 'Computer-aided drug design'(BP 807ET) in VIIIth semester. The main aim of this subject is to make students understand the process of drug discovery and development from the identification of drug targets to the introduction of new drugs.

The book *Computer-Aided Drug Design,* written in an easy to understand language, has been compiled in 11 chapters and appendices. The book is supplemented with well-illustrated figures, tables, appendices, etc. At the end, question bank is added to recapitulate the basics and help students prepare for their semester examination.

We hope that this book will definitely help students as well as the teachers alike. Constructive suggestions and comments on this book are most welcome.

We are thankful to Mr SK Jain (CMD), CBS Publishers & Distributors, New Delhi, for bringing out this book in the present form.

Anees Ahmad Siddiqui
Harish Kumar
Subuhi Khisal

Contents

Syllabus

BP 807 ET.   **COMPUTER-AIDED DRUG DESIGN (Theory)**

Scope: This subject is designed to provide detailed knowledge of rational drug design process and various techniques used in rational drug design process

Objectives: Upon completion of the course, the student shall be able to understand design and discovery of lead molecules
- The role of drug design in drug discovery process
- The concept of QSAR and docking
- Various strategies to develop new drug like molecules
- The design of new drug molecules using molecular modeling software

Course Content

UNIT I

Introduction to drug discovery and development stages of drug discovery and development

Lead discovery and analog based drug design rational approaches to lead discovery based on traditional medicine, random screening, non-random screening, serendipitous drug discovery, lead discovery based on drug metabolism, lead discovery based on clinical observation

Analog based drug design: Bioisosterism, classification, bioisosteric replacement [any three case studies]

UNIT II

Quantitative structure–activity relationship (QSAR) SAR *versus* QSAR, history and development of QSAR, types of physicochemical parameters, experimental and theoretical approaches for the determination of physicochemical parameters such as partition coefficient, Hammet's substituent constant and Tafts steric constant. Hansch analysis, Free Wilson analysis, 3D-QSAR approaches like CoMFA and CoMSIA

UNIT III

Molecular modeling and virtual screening techniques

Virtual screening techniques: Drug likeness screening, concept of pharmacophore mapping and pharmacophore based screening

Molecular docking: Rigid docking, flexible docking, manual docking, docking based screening, de novo drug design

UNIT IV

Informatics and methods in drug design, introduction to bioinformatics, chemoinformatics. ADME databases, chemical, biochemical and pharmaceutical databases

UNIT V

Molecular Modeling: Introduction to molecular mechanics and quantum mechanics. Energy minimization methods and conformational analysis, global conformational minima determination.

Acronyms

ADMET: Absorption, Distribution, Metabolism, Excretion and Toxicity

AFMoC: Adaptation of Fields for Molecular comparison

ANN: Artificial Neural Networks

CADD: Computer-Aided Drug Design

CASD: Computer-Assisted Synthesis Design

CASE: Computer-Assisted Structure Elucidation

CoMFA: Comparative Molecular Field Analysis

CoMSIA: Comparative Molecular Similarity Indices Analysis

CoRIA: Comparative Residue Interaction Analysis

COMBINE: Comparative Binding Energy Analysis

CoMSA: Comparative Molecular Surface Analysis

CoMMA: Comparative Molecular Moment Analysis

CoRSA: Comparative Receptor Surface Analysis

C- QSAR: Comparative Quantitative Structure–Activity Relationship

DCGI: Drug Controller General of India

DTAB: Drugs Technical Advisory Board

EVA: Evaluation of a Novel Infrared Range Vibration-Based Descriptor

GEAC: Genetic Engineering Approval Committee

GERM: Genetically Evolved Receptor Model

GFA: Genetic Function Approximation

GLP: Good Laboratory Practices

GRIND: Grid Independent Molecular Descriptor

HASL: Hypothetical Active Site Lattice

HTS: High-Throughput Screening

H-QSAR: Hologram Quantitative Structure–Activity Relationship

IND: Investigational New Drug

kNN: k-nearest neighbour

LOO: Leave One Out

LFER: Linear Free-Energy Relationship

LR: Linear Regression

MM: Molecular Mechanics

MLR: Multiple Linear Regression

MSA: Molecular Shape Analysis

NDA: New Drug Application

PLS: Partial Least-Squares

PCS: Principal Component Analysis

PCR: Principal Component Regression

PLP: Piecewase Linear Potential

PMF: Potential of Mean Force

QM: Quantum Mechanics

QPLS: Quadratic Partial Least Squares

QSAR: Quantitative Structure–Activity Relationship

QSPR: Quantitative Structure–Property Relationship

RIPS: Random Incremental Pulse Search

SAR: Structure–Activity Relationships

SoMFA: Self organising Molecular Field Analysis

SUMM: Systematic Unbounded Minimum Method

WHIM: Weight Holistic Invariant Molecular Indices

1 | Drug Discovery and Stages of Drug Development

INTRODUCTION

Drug discovery and development process starts with the aim to make available new pharmacological interventions to prevent, treat, mitigate, or cure disease in a safe and effective manner. Presently, it is mainly focused to treat cancer, diabetes, AIDS, infectious diseases, *etc*. The development of new drugs is very complex, costly and risky. Its success is highly dependent on an intense collaboration and interaction between several departments within the drug development organization, external investigators and service providers, in constant dialogue with regulatory authorities, payers, academic experts, clinicians and patient organizations. Within the different phases of the drug life cycle, drug development is by far the most crucial part for the initial and continued success of a drug on the market. Drug development starts with a target identification and validation, followed by drug candidates (hits) discovery, and lead drug (compound with favorable pharmaceutical, safety, efficacy, and pharmacokinetic profile) selection and optimization. Preclinical (non clinical) efficacy, pharmacology, toxicology, and mechanistic studies may include *in silico* (computational) methods, use of *in vitro* animal or human tissues (including cells and subcellular fractions), and *in vivo* animals. The studies rely on models that are thought to be predictive of the subsequent preclinical or clinical effects.

Drug development process proceeds through several stages in order to produce a product that is safe, efficacious, and has passed all regulatory requirements.

STAGE 1: DISCOVERY AND DEVELOPMENT

Discovery

Typically, researchers discover new drugs through:

Target identification: Drug discovery often begins with target identification. Ideally, the target should be the cause of a specific disease which can be targeted on a molecular level. Choosing a biochemical mechanism involved in a disease condition may be a target or particular receptor system may be a target. The human body functions normally by the virtue of the biochemical process which goes, producing all the necessary chemicals required for numerous functions to undergo smoothly within the body. Many of these processes are regulated by the enzymes and the endogenous effect or molecules via their respective receptors. A diseased state, may hence, be identified by, either the abnormal biochemical functioning or, over or underproduction of some of the intermediates. Hence, the most important and most common biological targets for drug discovery are either enzymes regulating the biochemistry or the receptors through which many hormones and endogenous effectors show their response. For example, inhibition of human dihydrofolate reductase, by methotrexate, brought under control the growth of tumor in humans. Similarly, blocking of the beta adrenoceptors in the cardiac muscles was found to reduce the hypertensive state. Another type of biological targets is nucleic acids. Though, they are rarely targeted as compared to those mentioned above, yet they are important targets.

Target validation: Once the target is identified, it becomes absolutely necessary to confirm, that the correct target has been identified. A crucial issue is to validate the target, in animals and preferably in human models. The use of reliable and suitable animal models and the latest techniques in gene targeting and expression are all essential to the validation process.

- Conduct of many tests of molecular compounds to find possible beneficial effects against any of a large number of existing diseases.
- Review of existing treatments that have unanticipated effects.
- New technologies, such as those that provide new ways to target medical products to specific sites within the body or to manipulate genetic material.

At this stage in the process, thousands of compounds may be potential candidates for development as a medical treatment. After early testing, however, only a small number of compounds look promising and selected for further study.

Identifying leads: A lead is a combination of molecules that is thought to have the capacity to treat disease. The lead retains elements required in the new medication. Clinical researchers assess already proven substances with the new combinations to evaluate their effectiveness. To verify the success of each molecule's effect on the drug target, clinical analysis is performed.

Optimizing leads: To assist biopharmaceutical companies choose the compound, or compounds, to be developed into safe and effective drugs, lead optimization compare the properties of various lead compounds with the highest probability of success.

Development

Once researchers identify a promising compound for development, they conduct experiments to gather information on:
- How it is absorbed, distributed, metabolized, and excreted (ADME of drug).
- Its potential benefits and mechanisms of action.
- The best dosage form (for example oral tablet or capsule, IV or IM injections).
- The best route of administration.
- Side effects or adverse events that can often be referred to as toxicity.
- How it affects different groups of people (such as by gender, race, or ethnicity) differently.
- How it interacts with other drugs and treatments.
- Its effectiveness as compared with similar drugs.

STAGE 2: PRECLINICAL RESEARCH

Preclinical trials, also known as non-clinical trials are the laboratory tests of a new drug, device or medical treatment on animal subjects or cell lines or enzymes. The main aim of preclinical studies is to see whether the drug or the treatment really works and

whether it is safe to test on humans. The preclinical studies are conducted on animal models under laboratory conditions. The two types of preclinical research are:
- *In vitro:* These are performed in test tube or elsewhere outside a living system.
- *In vivo:* These experiments are performed inside living organism.

The various experiments conducted during these studies include:

Acute Toxicity Studies

Acute toxicity studies look at the effects of one or more doses administered over a period of 24 hours. The goal is to determine toxic dose levels and observe clinical indications of toxicity. Usually, at least two mammalian species are tested. Data from acute toxicity studies helps to determine doses for repeated dose studies in animals and Phase I studies in humans.

Repeated Dose Studies

This comprises the adverse general toxicological effect. Depending on the duration of the study, repeated dose studies may be referred to as sub acute, sub chronic, or chronic. The specific duration should anticipate the length of the clinical trial that will be conducted on the new drug. Again, two species are typically required.

Pharmacological Studies for Safety Profile

It's a simple and rapidly performed initial screening test to determine the presence or absence of a particular pharmacodynamic activity in the new drug, e.g. determination of analgesic or pain relieving activity in the new drug. Besides determination of the action of the drug, its effects on individual and major organ systems like nervous, cardio-vascular, respiratory, and renal are also examined. This can give a clue about any possible side-effects of the drug on any major organ system.

Genotoxicity Studies

These studies assess the mutagenic or carcinogenic properties of drug. Procedures such as the Ames test (conducted in bacteria) detect genetic changes. DNA damage is assessed in tests using mammalian cells such as the Mouse Micronucleus Test. The Chromosomal Aberration Test and similar procedures detect damage at the chromosomal level.

Carcinogenicity Studies

Carcinogenicity studies are usually needed only for drugs intended for chronic or recurring conditions. They are time consuming and expensive, and must be planned for early in the preclinical testing process. They may be needed to support marketing approval of some botanical drug.

Reproductive Toxicity Studies

Segment I reproductive toxicity studies look at the effects of the drug on fertility. Segment II and III studies detect effects on embryonic and post-natal development. In general, reproductive toxicity studies must be completed before a drug can be administered to women of child-bearing age.

FDA requires researchers to use good laboratory practices (GLP), defined in medical product development regulations, for preclinical laboratory studies. The GLP regulations are set the minimum basic requirements for:

- study conduct
- personnel
- facilities
- equipment
- written protocols
- operating procedures
- study reports
- and a system of quality assurance oversight for each study to help assure the safety of FDA-regulated product

STAGE 3: CLINICAL RESEARCH

While preclinical research answers basic questions about a drug's safety, it is not a substitute for studies of ways; the drug will interact with the human body. "Clinical research" refers to studies, or trials, that are done on humans. As the developers design the clinical study, they will consider what they want to accomplish for each of the different clinical research phases and begin the investigational new drug process (IND), a process they must go through before clinical research begins.

Designing Clinical Trials

Researchers design clinical trials to answer specific research questions related to a medical product. These trials follow a specific study plan, called a protocol, which is developed by the researcher or manufacturer. Before a clinical trial begins, researchers review prior information about the drug to develop research questions and objectives. Then, they decide:

- Who qualifies to participate (selection criteria)
- How many people will be part of the study
- How long the study will last
- Whether there will be a control group and other ways to limit research bias
- How the drug will be given to patients and at what dosage
- What assessments will be conducted, when, and what data will be collected
- How the data will be reviewed and analyzed

Clinical trials follow a typical series from early, small-scale, Phase 1 studies to late-stage, large scale, Phase 3 studies.

Clinical Research Phase Studies

Clinical trials are the way to test new methods of diagnosing, treating or preventing health conditions. The goal is to determine whether something is both safe and effective.

Phase 0 (Microdosing) – Phase '0' of a clinical trial is done with a very small number of people, usually fewer than 15. Investigator uses a small dose of medication to make sure, it is not harmful to humans before they start using it in higher doses for later phases.

Phase 1 (First in Humans) – In this phase, testing of drug on healthy volunteers is done for dose adjustments.

Trial Design

Patients: 20 to 100 healthy volunteers or people with the disease/condition.

Duration of study: Short—Days to several weeks or months

Type of study: Open label (no placebo or comparative agent), uncontrolled, single or multiple doses.

Purpose (intended for knowing the safety and dosage) including:-

- Mechanism of action (ADME) and PK/PD studies
- Pharmacological effect
- Tolerability, side effects and toxicity at different doses
- Early evidence of efficacy
- Evaluates safety – Identify most likely potential toxicities and most likely dosage range **approximately 70% of drugs move to the next phase.**

Phase 2 (Therapeutic Exploratory) – In this phase, testing of drug is performed on patients to assess efficacy and adverse effects.

Trial Design

Patients: Several hundred (100-300) patients with the targeted disease/condition.

Length of Study: Several months to 2 years

Purpose: Efficacy and side effects

Type of study: Randomized, placebo or active control, parallel double blinded study, single or multiple doses, multicenter.

Purpose

- Dose range finding (minimum and maximum effective dose).
- Effectiveness for the treatment of the disease or condition for which the drug is intended to use
- Maximum tolerated dose (MTD)
- Common short time side effects and risks
- Pharmacokinetics

The percentage of drugs that move to the next phase is 33%.

Phase 3 (Therapeutic Confirmatory) – Pivotal Trials – Trials on patients are performed to assess efficacy, safety and effectiveness of the drug under investigation at large scale.

Trial Design

Patients: Several 1000 to 3,000 patients with the targeted disease/condition.

Length of Study: 1 to 4 years

Type of study: Randomized, placebo or active control, parallel double blinded study, multicenter

Purpose

- Effectiveness (Large scale)
- Relative risk/benefit relationship

- Long term safety information – common side effects, drug interactions, age/rate/gender differences
- Dosing (for labeling)
- Assessment of safety and efficacy

Percentage of drugs that move to the next phase is 25–30%.

After completing the phase III trail the application is filed with the concerned regulatory bodies seeking permission for marketing and after the regulatory bodies grant the required approval, the product is launched into the market.

Phase 4 (Post-marketing Therapeutic Use) – This investigation takes place on the new marketed drug which is approved by the FDA. This phase involves thousands of participants and can last for many years.

Trial Design

Patients: Several hundred to thousand patients with the disease/condition.

Type of study: Randomized, Placebo or active control, Multicenter

Purpose

- Perform Quality of Life Trails (QOL) trails
- Perform pharmacoeconomic trails – Is the drug more effective that other available treatments
- Collection of long term safety information – Epidemiological studies for safety and additional surveillance for unexpected or rare adverse effects
- Add line extensions – New dosage forms and formulations

The Investigational New Drug Process

Drug developers, or sponsors, must submit an Investigational New Drug (IND) application to FDA before beginning clinical research.

In the IND application, developers must include:

- Animal study data and toxicity (side effects that cause great harm) data
- Manufacturing information
- Clinical protocols (study plans) for studies to be conducted
- Data from any prior human research
- Information about the investigator

Asking for FDA Assistance

Drug developers are free to ask for help from FDA at any point in the drug development process, including:

- Pre-IND application, to review FDA guidance documents and get answers to questions that may help enhance their research
- After Phase 2, to obtain guidance on the design of large Phase 3 studies
- Any time during the process, to obtain an assessment of the IND application

Even though FDA offers extensive technical assistance, drug developers are not required to take FDA's suggestions. As long as clinical trials are thoughtfully designed, reflect what developers know about a product, safeguard participants, and otherwise meet Federal standards, FDA allows wide latitude in clinical trial design.

FDA IND Review Team

The review team consists of a group of specialists in different scientific fields. Each member has different responsibilities.

- *Project Manager:* Coordinates the team's activities throughout the review process, and is the primary contact for the sponsor.
- *Medical Officer:* Reviews all clinical study information and data before, during, and after the trial is complete.
- *Statistician:* Interprets clinical trial designs and data, and works closely with the medical officer to evaluate protocols and safety and efficacy data.
- *Pharmacologist:* Reviews preclinical studies.
- *Pharmakineticist:* Focuses on the drug's absorption, distribution, metabolism, and excretion processes. Interprets blood-level data at different time intervals from clinical trials, as a way to assess drug dosages and administration schedules.
- *Chemist:* Evaluates a drug's chemical compounds. Analyzes how a drug was made and its stability, quality control, continuity, the presence of impurities, *etc.*
- *Microbiologist:* Reviews the data submitted, if the product is an antimicrobial product, to assess response across different classes of microbes.

Approval

The FDA review team has 30 days to review the original IND submission. The process protects volunteers who participate in clinical trials from unreasonable and significant risk in clinical trials. FDA responds to IND applications in one of two ways:

- Approval to begin clinical trials.
- Clinical hold to delay or stop the investigation. FDA can place a clinical hold for specific reasons, including:
  - o Participants are exposed to unreasonable or significant risk.
  - o Investigators are not qualified.
  - o Materials for the volunteer participants are misleading.
  - o The IND application does not include enough information about the trial's risks.

A clinical hold is rare; instead, FDA often provides comments intended to improve the quality of a clinical trial. In most cases, if FDA is satisfied that the trial meets Federal standards, the applicant is allowed to proceed with the proposed study.

The developer is responsible for informing the review team about new protocols, as well as serious side effects seen during the trial. This information ensures that the team can monitor the trials carefully for signs of any problems. After the trial ends, researchers must submit study reports.

This process continues until the developer decides to end clinical trials or files a marketing application. Before filing a marketing application, a developer must have adequate data from two large, controlled clinical trials.

STAGE 4: FDA DRUG REVIEW

If a drug developer has evidence from its early tests and preclinical and clinical research that a drug is safe and effective for its intended use, the company can file an application to market the drug. The FDA review team thoroughly examines all submitted data on the drug and makes a decision to approve or not to approve it.

New Drug Application

A new drug application (NDA) tells the full story of a drug. Its purpose is to demonstrate that a drug is safe and effective for its intended use in the population studied.

A drug developer must include everything about a drug—from preclinical data to Phase 3 trial data—in an NDA. Developers must include reports on all studies, data, and analyses. Along with clinical results, developers must include:
- Proposed labeling
- Safety updates
- Drug abuse information
- Patent information
- Any data from studies that may have been conducted outside the United States
- Institutional review board compliance information
- Directions for use

FDA Review

Once FDA receives an NDA, the review team decides if it is complete. If it is not complete, the review team can refuse to file the NDA. If it is complete, the review team has 6 to 10 months to make a decision on whether to approve the drug. The process includes the following:
- Each member of the review team conducts a full review of his or her section of the application. For example, the medical officer and the statistician review clinical data, while a pharmacologist reviews the data from animal studies. Within each technical discipline represented on the team, there is also a supervisory review.
- FDA inspectors travel to clinical study sites to conduct a routine inspection. The Agency looks for evidence of fabrication, manipulation, or withholding of data.
- The project manager assembles all individual reviews and other documents, such as the inspection report, into an "action package." This document becomes the record for FDA review. The review team issues a recommendation, and a senior FDA official makes a decision.

FDA Approval

In cases where FDA determines that a drug has been shown to be safe and effective for its intended use, it is then necessary to work with the applicant to develop and refine prescribing information. This is referred to as "labeling." Labeling accurately and objectively describes the basis for approval and how best to use the drug.

Often, though, remaining issues need to be resolved before the drug can be approved for marketing. Sometimes FDA requires the developer to address questions based on existing data. In other cases, FDA requires additional studies. At this point, the developer can decide whether or not to continue further development. If a developer disagrees with an FDA decision, there are mechanisms for formal appeal.

FDA Advisory Committees

Often, the NDA contains sufficient data for FDA to determine the safety and effectiveness of a drug. Sometimes, though, questions arise that require additional consideration. In these cases, FDA may organize a meeting of one of its Advisory

Committees to get independent, expert advice and to permit the public to make comments. These Advisory Committees include a Patient Representative that provides input from the patient perspective. Learn more about FDA Advisory Committees.

STAGE 5: FDA POST-MARKET DRUG SAFETY MONITORING

Even though clinical trials provide important information on a drug's efficacy and safety, it is impossible to have complete information about the safety of a drug at the time of approval. Despite the rigorous steps in the process of drug development, limitations exist. Therefore, the true picture of a product's safety actually evolves over the months and even years that make up a product's lifetime in the marketplace. FDA reviews reports of problems with prescription and over-the-counter drugs, and can decide to add cautions to the dosage or usage information, as well as other measures for more serious issues.

FDA Post-market drug safety monitoring includes:
- Supplemental applications
- INDs for marketed drugs
- Manufacturer inspections
- Drug advertising
- Generic drugs
- Reporting problems
- Active surveillance

Supplemental Applications

Developers must file a supplemental application if they wish to make any significant changes from the original NDA. Generally, any changes in formulation, labeling, or dosage strength must be approved by FDA before they can be made.

INDs for Marketed Drugs

If sponsors want to further develop an approved drug for a new use, dosage strength, new form, or different form (such as an injectable or oral liquid, as opposed to tablet form), or if they want to conduct other clinical research or a post-market safety study, they would do so under an IND.

Manufacturer Inspections

FDA officials conduct routine inspections of drug manufacturing facilities across the United States, and abroad if approved products are manufactured overseas. Manufacturers may be informed of inspections in advance, or the inspections may be unannounced. Inspections may be routine or caused by a particular problem or concern. The purpose of these inspections is to make sure that developers are following good manufacturer practice. FDA can shut down a facility if minimum standards are not met.

Drug Advertising*

FDA regulates prescription drug advertisements and promotional labeling. By law, a developer is prohibited from advertising unapproved uses of their product.

---

* Learn more at prescription drug advertising.

All advertisements, such as product claims or reminder ads, cannot be false or misleading. They must contain truthful information about a drug's effectiveness, side effects, and prescribing information. These advertisements can be found in medical journals, newspapers, and magazines, and on the Internet, television, or radio.

Promotional labeling differs from drug advertisements in the way it is distributed. Pharmaceutical companies give out brochures or other promotional materials to physicians or consumers. The drug's prescribing information must accompany promotional labeling.

Generic Drugs

A generic drug is pharmaceutical drug having some chemical substance as originally developed and patented drug. Generic drugs are allowed for sale after patent on original drug expires. New drugs are patent protected when they are approved for marketing. This means that only the sponsor has the right to market the drug exclusively. Once the patent expires, other drug manufacturers can develop the drug, which will be known as a generic version of the drug for example: Metformin is the generic name for which a brand name is Glucophage. Generic drugs are comparable to brand name drugs and must have the same:

- Dosage form
- Strength
- Safety
- Quality
- Performance characteristics
- Intended use

Because generic drugs are comparable to drugs already on the market, generic drug manufacturers do not have to conduct clinical trials to demonstrate that their product is safe and effective. Instead, they conduct bio-equivalence studies and file an abbreviated new drug application.

Indian Scenario

Demonstration of safety and efficacy of the drug product for use in humans is essential before the drug product can be approved for manufacturing/import. Manufacturing, importing or conducting a clinical trial requires permission from licensing authority, Central Drugs Standard Control Organization (CDSCO) through a Form 44 application (Table 1.1). This organization has six zonal offices, four sub-zonal offices, 13 port offices, and seven laboratories under its control. The regulations under Drugs and Cosmetics Act 1940 and its rules 1945, 122A, 122B and 122D and further Appendix I, IA and VI of Schedule Y, describe the information required for approval of an application to manufacture of new drug for marketing. Through the International Conference on Harmonization (ICH) process, the Common Technical Document (CTD) guidance has been developed for Japan, European Union, and United States. Most countries have adopted the CTD format. Hence, CDSCO has also decided to adopt CTD format for technical requirements for registration of pharmaceutical products for human use. It is apparent that this structured application with comprehensive and rational contents will help the CDSCO to review and take necessary actions in a better way and would also ease the preparation of electronic submissions, which may happen in the near future at CDSCO.

Form No. and Rules	Purpopse
44	Application for permission to import or manufacture a new drug or to begin a new clinical trial
122-A	Application for permission to import a new drug
122-B	Application for approval to import a new drug
122-D	Permission to import or manufacture fixed dose combination
122-DA	Application for permission to conduct a clinical trial for new drug or investigational new drug
122-DAA	Definition of clinical trial
122-DB	Suspension or cancellation of permission or approval

Table 1.1: New drug application forms and rules

Drug Controller General of India

Clinical Research is regulated in India by Drug Controller General of India (DCGI). The office of DCGI runs under CDSCO. It has main responsibility of regulating clinical trials in India. Permission is necessary from DCGI through Form no 44. Matters related to product approval and standards, clinical trials, introduction of new drug, and import licenses of new drugs are handled by DCGI.

Drugs Technical Advisory Board (DTAB): It has technical experts and this advice the central and state governments on all technical matters arising out of the enforcement of drug control. No rules can be made by the central government without consulting DTAB board.

Drugs Consultative Committee: It has central and state drug control officials as members. Its main function is to ensure the drug control measures and enforce them uniformly over all the states.

Genetic Engineering approval Committee (GEAC): It is authority to approve r-DNA (recombinant DNA) pharmaceuticals products. GEAC's role is to assess the bio-safety/environmental safety aspect of the biotechnological product.

2

Lead Discovery and Drug Design

The term' drug design' is referred to development of new drug on rational basis. There are various approaches like random screening of synthetic compounds, synthesis of biologically active compounds based on naturally occurring drug, synthesis of structural analogues of naturally occurring lead compounds and application of bioisosteric principle. Thus, in the current trend, drug design involves either total innovation of lead or an optimization of already available lead. A lead compound is also called as leading compound. The lead is a prototype compound that has the desired biological or pharmacological activity but may also have many undesirable characteristics like high toxicity, other biological activities (side effects), insolubility or metabolism problems and once identified, are easy to exploit. This process is rather straight forward. The real task lies in the identification of such lead compound and the optimum bioactive positions on the basic skeleton of such leads.

SERENDIPITOUS DRUG DISCOVERY

The examples of drug discovery without a lead structure are very few in number. These include the serendipitous discoveries. In *Stedman's medical dictionary* "serendipity" refers to "an accidental discovery" means, "finding one thing while looking for something else". Serendip is a former name for Sri Lanka. The three princes made their discoveries "by accident and sagacity", according to Walpole.

The story begins in 1856 with an 18-year-old English chemist named William Henry Perkins (1838–1907), who was trying to synthesize quinine and ended up with a bluish substance that he extracted from a "black mass" in his test tube, which had excellent dyeing properties. Perkins' discovery of the first artificial dye in history, variably referred to as aniline purple, tyrian blue or mauve, triggered a chain reaction by serendipity. Modifications of his process led to the development of many dyes and the emergence of the dye industry (Bayer in 1862, Ciba in 1859, Geigy in 1859, and Sandoz in 1862).

Some other examples of remarkable serendipitous drug discoveries are presented in this chapter.

Penicillin

Fleming was engaged in research on influenza when one of his staphylococcus culture plates had become contaminated and developed a mold that created a bacteria-free circle. Fleming recognized the possible significance of the bacteria-free circle, and by isolating the mold in pure culture he found that it produced a substance that has a powerful destructive effect on many of the common bacteria that infect man. He named the antibacterial substance liberated into the fluid in which the mold was grown "penicillin", after *Penicillium notatum*, the contaminant of the staphylococcus colony that led to the discovery.

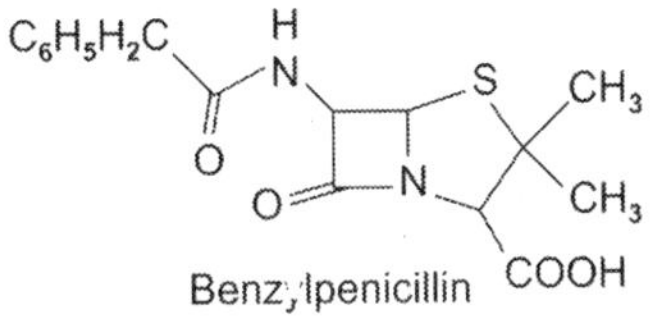

Benzylpenicillin 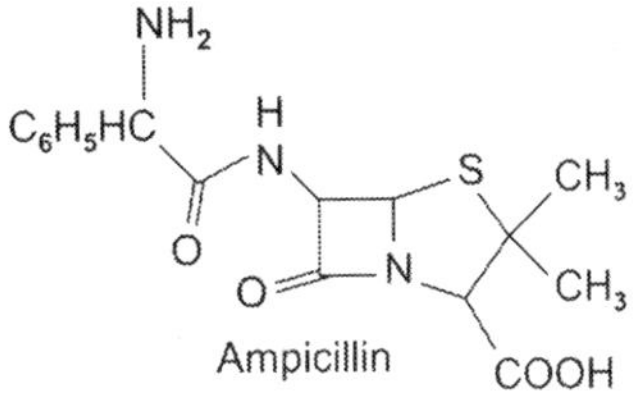   Ampicillin

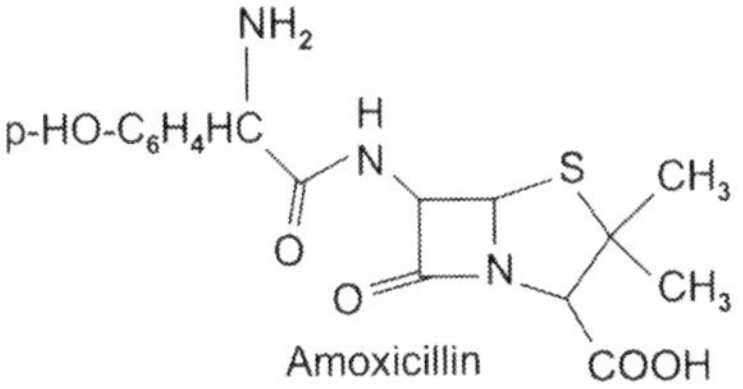

Amoxicillin

Although, Fleming published his results in the *Journal of Experimental Pathology* in 1929, it was only 10 years later that Howard Florey and his team embarked on the research that culminated in 1941 in the development of a methodology for the extraction and production of penicillin. To obtain sufficient, quantity of the substance for clinical use, the original strain, *Penicillium notatum*, had to be replaced by *Penicillium chrysogenum*. Two years later, John Mahoney and his associates in the US Public Health Service, demonstrated that penicillin was highly effective in the treatment of primary syphilis; and in 1944, Stokes and his associates at Johns Hopkins hospital in Baltimore, Maryland, reported on the therapeutic effect of penicillin in the treatment, of "late syphilis including neurosyphilis". Since neurosyphilis and infectious delirium represented a considerable proportion of psychiatric patients, by changing the diagnostic distribution of patients, the introduction of penicillin resulted in a shift in priorities in psychiatric research from the "organic" to the "functional" psychiatric disorders by the end of the 1940.

The correct structure was reported in 1943 by Sir Robirtson and Karl Folkers. Once, the structure was known, it became the lead nucleus for future more effective analogues-ampicillin, amoxicillin, *etc*.

Chlordiazepoxide (Librium)

Librium (tranquilizer drug) is an another example of drug, discovered without a lead. A series of quinazoline-3-oxides was synthesized by Leo Sternbatch at Roche to develop a new class of tranquilizer drugs. Since none of these compounds was found to be active and so the scheme was terminated in 1955.

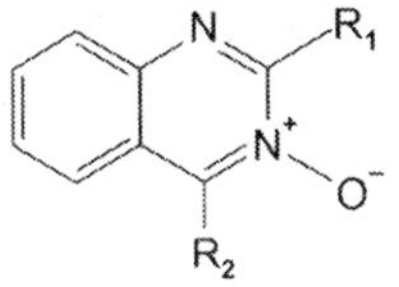

Quinazoline-3-oxide

However, a vial from the above scheme which remained untested was found in 1957 during a general laboratory cleanup. The compound (**A**) supposed to be present in it, was submitted for pharmacological testing, to complete official formalities. Surprisingly, it gave promising results. It was found due to benzodiazine-4-oxide, probably produced in an unexpected reaction of the corresponding chloromethyl quinazoline-3-oxide with methylamine. It was named, Librium. This drug, Librium (lead compound) was exploited to develop future analogs like oxazepam, diazepam, *etc.*

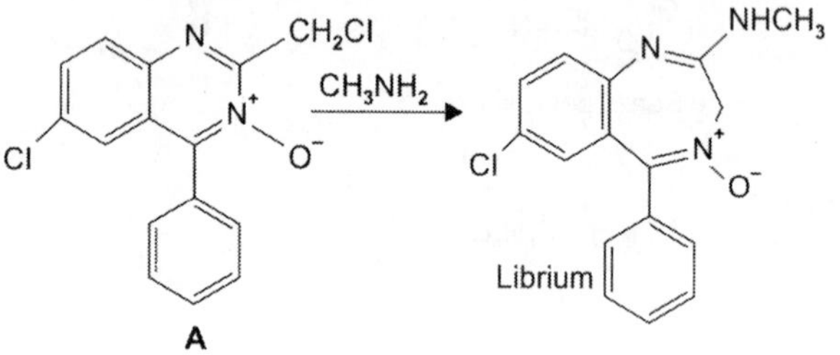

A

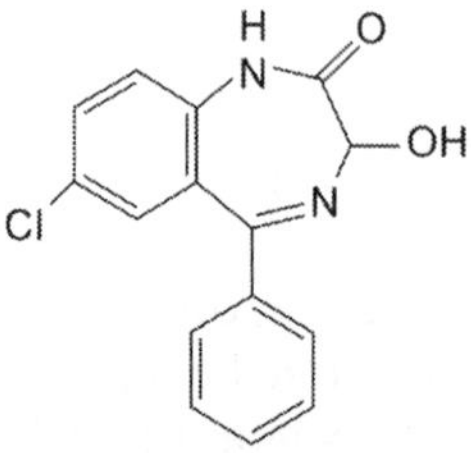

Librium

Oxazepam 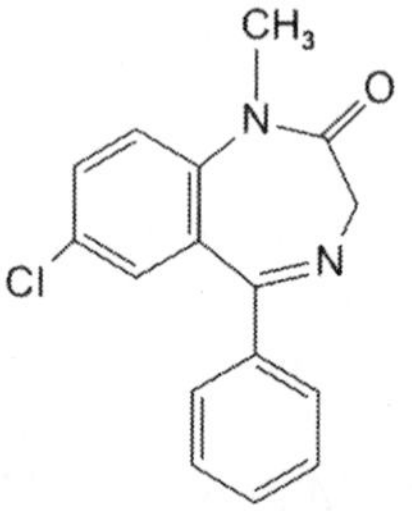   Diazepam

Warfarin

The event leading to the discovery of Warfarin started in the early 20th century by the reports of deaths of cattle in the United States and Canada due to severe internal bleeding. In 1922, a specialist in veterinary medicine, Schofield, postulated that these deaths were being caused by the cattle eating spoiled sweet clover hay. Only spoiled hay made from sweet clover (grown in northern states of the USA and in Canada since the turn of the century) produced the disease. Schofield separated good clover stalks and damaged clover stalks from the same hay mow, and fed each to a different rabbit. The rabbit that had ingested the good stalks remained well, but the rabbit that had ingested the damaged stalks died from a hemorrhagic illness. It was a mystery as to why this spoilt sweet clover hay had these effects until 1939 when Karl Paul Link and his team at the University of Wisconsin discovered the compound that had caused these effects. It was dicoumarol. This compound was formed from the oxidation of coumarin, which is in fresh sweet clover hay, by fungi in the spoilt hay. Dicoumarol was used as an oral anticoagulant once its' effects had been discovered.

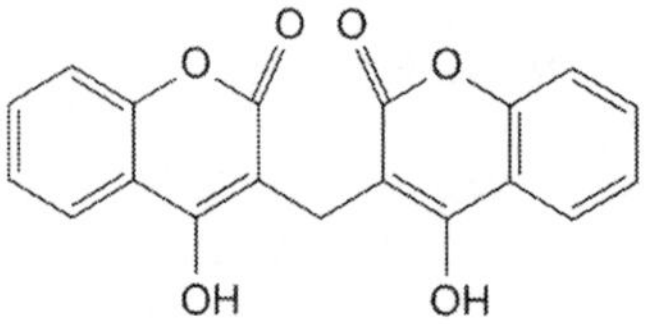

Dicoumarol 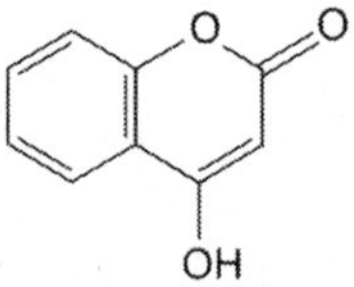   Coumarin

Interest was regenerated after the Second World War when in 1946 Link and his team turned their attentions to the development of a rat poison. Dicoumarol was ineffective as a rodenticide and they later discovered, 3-phenylacetyl ethyl 4-hydroxycoumarin, which was a very potent rodenticide and patents rights were assigned to the **Wisconsin Alumni Research Foundation**. This lead to the name **WARFARIN**. In 1948, Warfarin was launched as the perfect rat poison.

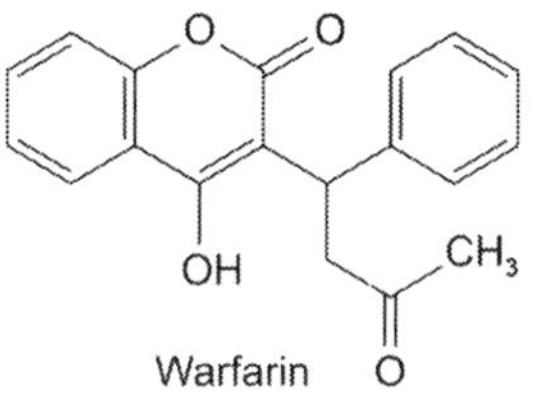

Warfarin

The first clinical study of Warfarin for use in humans was carried out in the early 1950's. This had been brought about due to a failed suicide attempt by a navy recruit who had tried to kill himself by taking an overdose of the rat poison, Warfarin. These studies had a great impact on the use of Warfarin and in 1955, Warfarin was even given to Eisenhower (American) following his heart attack.

Nitrous Oxide (N_2O)

Nitrous oxide, or laughing gas was discovered in 1772 by English Clergyman and scientist Joseph Priestly (the man who also the first to isolate oxygen, carbon monoxide and carbon dioxide). Priestly found that putting iron fillings into nitric acid released the gas, which had antipanic properties. But it wasn't until the 1840s, when forward-thinking doctors and dentists began experimenting with it as a tranquilizer. In between, it had mainly been used as a mood enhancer at parties, and had gained a reputation as something of a recreational drug.

Cisplatin

It is well know that serendipity has played a pivotal role in the discovery of many drugs used today. Indeed two major classes of anticancer drugs were discovered with the aid of serendipity.

The discovery of cisplatin was serendipitous. In 1965, Rosenberg was looking into the effects of an electric field on the growth of *Escherichia coli* bacteria. He noticed that bacteria ceased to divide when placed in an electric field but what Rosenberg also observed was a 300-fold increase in the size of the bacteria. He attributed this to the fact that somehow the platinum-conducting plates were inducing cell growth but inhibiting cell division. It was later deduced that the platinum species responsible for this was cisplatin. Rosenberg hypothesized that if cisplatin could inhibit bacterial cell division it could also stop tumor cell growth. This conjecture has proven correct and has led to the introduction of cisplatin in cancer therapy. Indeed, in 1978, six years after clinical trials conducted by the NCI and Bristol-Myers-Squibb, the US Food and Drug Administration (FDA) approved cisplatin under the name of Platinol for treating patients with metastatic testicular or ovarian cancer in combination with other drugs but also for treating bladder cancer.

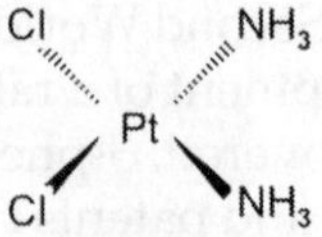

Cisplatin

With the discovery of cisplatin and the breakthrough observation by Lieutenant Colonel Stewart F Alexander, regarding the depletion of WBC by the chemical warfare agent, nitrogen mustard led to the development of alkylation agents.

Saccharin

In the 1870s, Russian chemist **Constantin Fahlberg** worked in the lab of Ira Remsen at Johns Hopkins University. Remsen's team experimented with coal-tar derivates, seeing how they react to phosphorus, chloride, ammonia, and other chemicals. One night, Fahlberg returned home and started to eat dinner rolls. The rolls tasted curiously sweet. The recipe hadn't changed, so what was going on here? He soon realized that it wasn't the rolls. It was him. His hands were covered with a mystery chemical that made everything sweet.

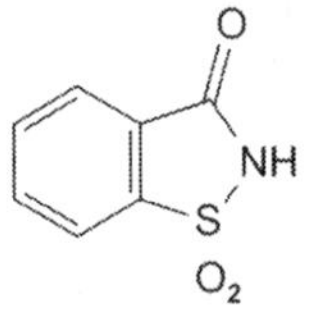

Saccharin

"Fahlberg had literally brought his work home with him, having spilled an experimental compound over his hands earlier that day," writes the Chemical Heritage Foundation in its history of saccharin. "He ran back to Remsen's laboratory, where he tasted everything on his worktable—all the vials, beakers, and dishes he used for his experiments. Finally he found the source: an overboiled beaker."

Fahlberg had actually created saccharin before, but since he never bothered to taste-test his concoctions, the chemist had no idea.

Lithium

In the mid-1800s, lithium was used to treat gout and bladder stones. After World War II, psychiatrist John Cade injected urine from healthy and mentally ill patients into the abdomens of guinea pigs. He found that the guinea pigs injected with urine from healthy patients died faster, which raised the idea that more uric acid was in the urine of the mentally ill patients.

In an attempt to increase the solubility of the uric acid, cade, added a lithium solution. Following injection, he noticed that the guinea pigs were sedated and calm rather than excited.

Interestingly, Cade ingested the lithium himself to ensure that it was safe for humans, and he later began administering it to patients with psychiatric disorders.

Methods of Lead Discovery

There are several approaches which can be adopted for identifying the lead structure. In order to identify a lead nucleus, in a given series, all compounds in a series should be tested for a particular biological activity. Once the lead is identified, it is modified to improve the potency. There is a difference between activity and potency. Activity is the particular pharmacological activity while potency is the strength of that effect. Various methods of lead identifications are as follows:

a. Random Screening

All the compounds (including synthetic and naturally occurring) from a given series are tested. In spite of more budgetary and manpower requirements, this method may be used to discover drugs or leads that have unexpected activities. Antibiotics like streptomycin and tetracycline were discovered by this method.

b. Nonrandom Screening

It is a modified form of random screening, developed to minimize the over budgetary and manpower requirement of random screening. In this method, only compounds having similar structural skeletons considering as lead are screened.

c. Drug Metabolism Studies

The metabolic biotransformation occurs with the help of enzymes to cut short the period of stay of drug in the body. The drug is structurally modified to increase the polarity to be more readily excreted out from body. It is done irrespective of the fact whether the resulting drug metabolites possess more activity or toxicity. The discovery of sulphanilamide is reported through the metabolic structures of prontosil (dye).

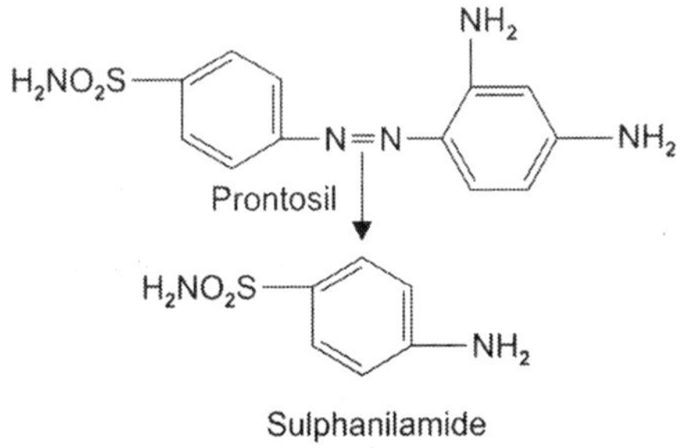

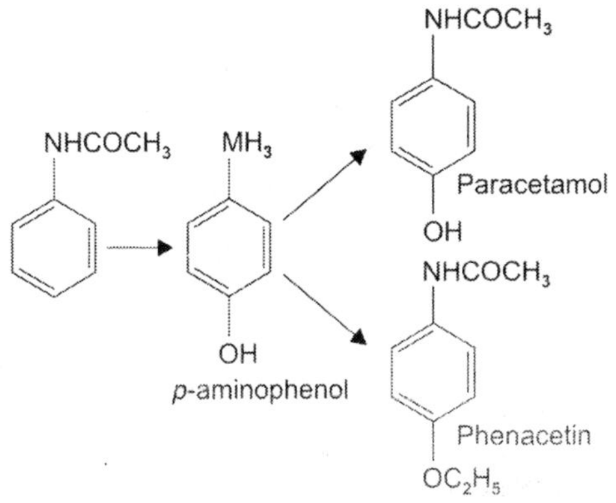

How, paracetamol is discovered; the antipyretic action of acetanilide was discovered by chance, when a nurse by mistake dispensed acetanilide to a patient. Due to its toxicities, it could not outstand in a market. Metabolic studies showed that toxicities are due to its *in vivo* metabolite, *p*-amino phenol. These observations led to development of phenacetin and paracetamol on chemical manipulation. Quite recently phenacetin has been withdrawn completely because of its toxic after effects, though it dominated the therapeutic field for over 30 years as a potent antipyretic and analgesics.

The study of the metabolite conversion of the antirheumatic drug phenylbutazone resulted in the introduction of a better tolerated drug oxyphenbutazone as an anti rheumatic drug and phenylbutazone alcohol as an uricosuric agent (substances that increase the excretion of uric acid in urine).

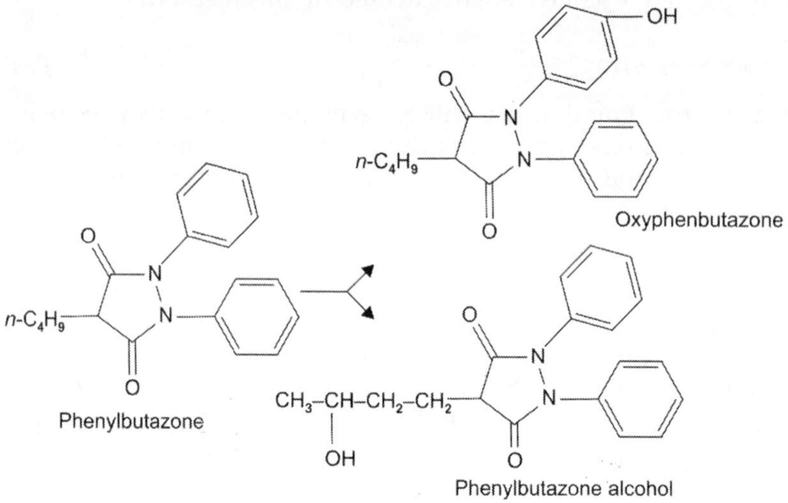

Oxyphenbutazone

Phenylbutazone

Phenylbutazone alcohol

More recently, the antihistaminic drug, cetrizine came in market, discovered on the basis of metabolic studies of hydroxyzine.

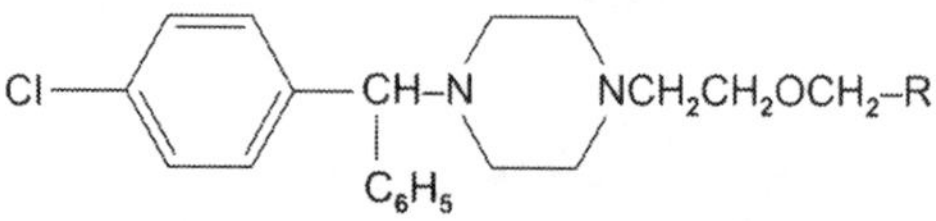

Hydroxyzine, R=COOH
Cetrizine, R=CH$_2$OH

Similarly, oxazepam finds the way in the clinical practice. It was observed to be metabolite of diazepam and found active.

d. Clinical Observations

Most of drugs possess more than one pharmacological activity. The main activity is called as *therapeutic effect* while other actions are known as side effects of drug. Such

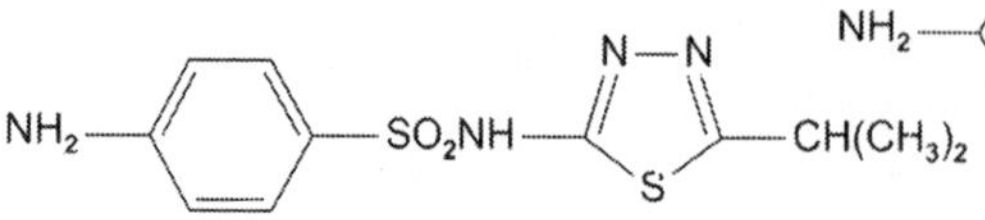

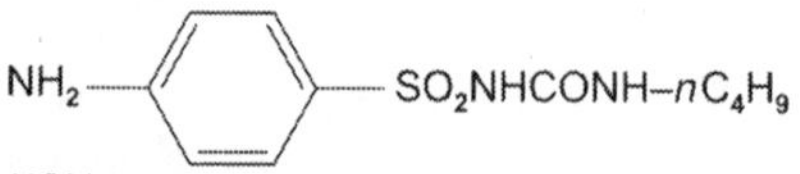

Carbutamide

5–isopropyl-2-sulphonamide-1,3,4–thiadiazole

drugs may be used as lead compounds for structural modifications to improve the potency of secondary effects.

The hypoglycemic sulphonylureas are developed from the clinical observations. In 1942, the sulphathiazole derivatives which were being used specifically for treating typhoid was observed to lower the blood glucose drastically. The pronounced hypoglycemic effect exerted by 5-isopropyl-2-sulphonamide– 1, 3, 4-thiadiazole indicated that an aryl sulphonyl thiourea moiety $(ArSO_2\text{-}NH\text{-}C\,(=N)\text{-}S)$ present in thiadiazole is responsible for their blood glucose lowering effect. This observation led to the development of carbutamide by Franke and Fukeks through the opening of thiazole ring of sulphathiazole to give a thiourea derivative in which =S was then replaced by =O group. In order to nullify the toxicity and antibacterial activity of *p*-amino group, it was replaced by other substituents resulting into tolbutamide, chlorpropamide, *etc.*

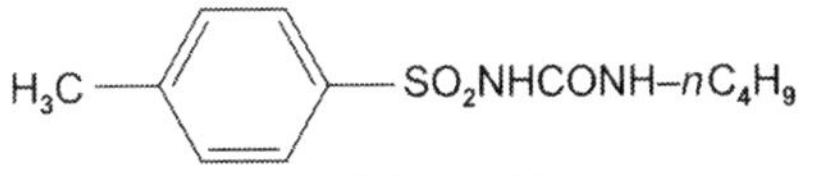

Tolbutamide 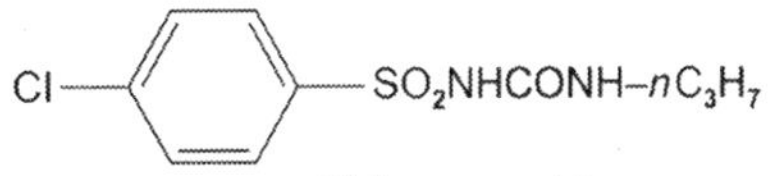   Chlorpropamide

In the 70s, the standard treatment for hypertension (high blood pressure) included beta blockers and diuretics, such as propranolol and hydrochlorothiazide, respectively. β-blockers possess many other different activities, including sedative and anti-convulsant effects. To enhance some of the secondary effects, the central core, or pharmacophore of beta blockers was modified to form a new ring (as shown below). A thorough study of derivatives of 'A' yielded the antidepressant, Viloxazine (Emovit). The research on viloxazine implies that different conformations of beta blockers are responsible for their poor target selectivity. Restriction of the flexibility by a standard method, tying the molecule with a ring, boosts selectivity for one of the targets.

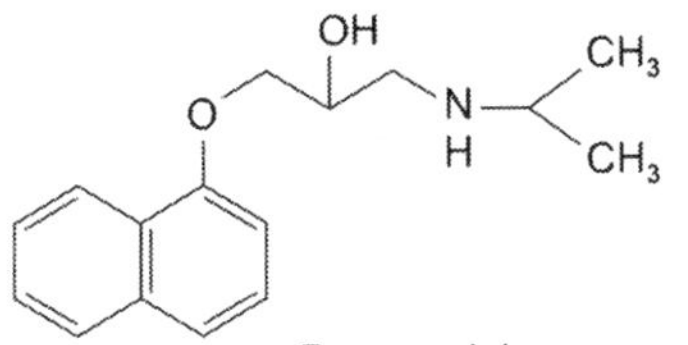

A   Propranalol 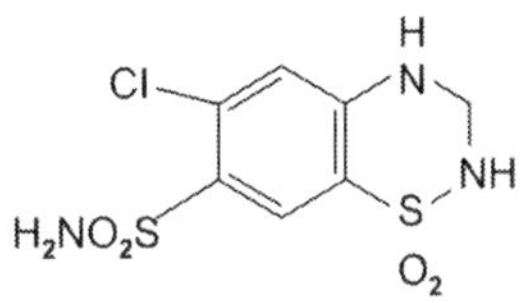   Hydrochlorothiazide

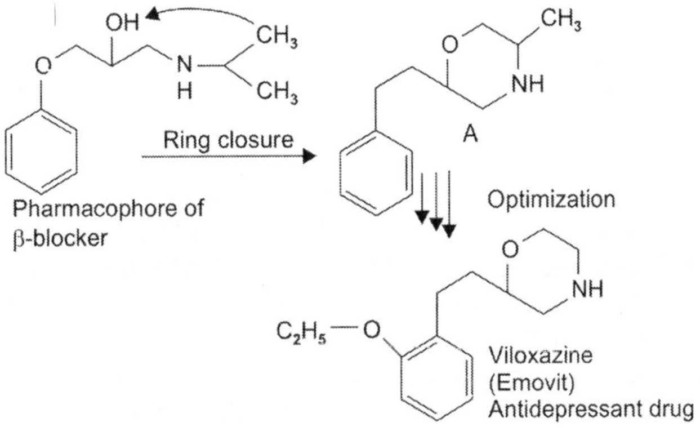

Pharmacophore of β-blocker

Ring closure

A

Optimization

Viloxazine (Emovit) Antidepressant drug

Viagra

In the late 1980s, a Pfizer research team in England developed a promising drug for treating angina, a condition characterized by tightness in the chest because of limited blood flow to the heart. The compound, known at the time as UK-92,480, entered clinical trials in healthy volunteers, the equivalent of Case Study–Phase I trials in the United States. Although UK-92,480 appeared to be safe, it had little impact on blood pressure, heart rate, and cardiac output. In a 1992 study, some volunteers receiving multiple doses reported an increased incidence of penile erections. Preliminary data was not overwhelming, but Pfizer spent another two years investigating the potential market for an erectile dysfunction drug. A study involving 300 patients in 1994 and 1995 showed excellent results for UK-92,480, which had been renamed sildenafil. The trials were so successful that, when the trials were complete, patients were reluctant to turn in their unused medication. Some patients even falsely claimed to have flushed leftover pills down the toilet in order to keep the unused medication. Sildenafil was approved by the FDA in early 1997 under the trade name Viagra. Despite competition in the marketplace from other erectile dysfunction drugs, Viagra has been a blockbuster for Pfizer, with a peak in sales of nearly US$2 billion worldwide in 2008.

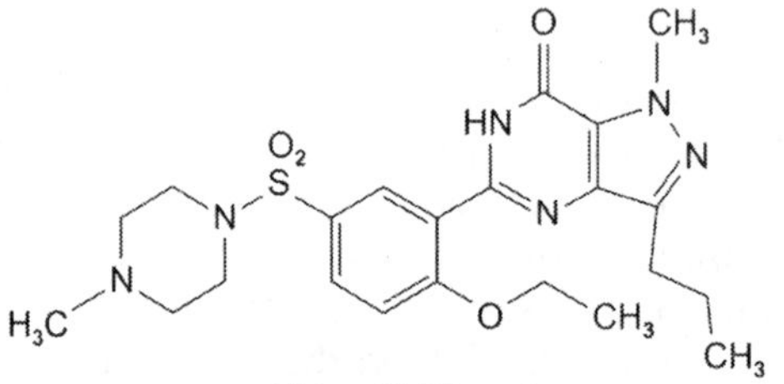

Sildenafil (Viagra)

Clonidine

It was initially discovered as nasal decongestant but it was found out that other effect were more significant. After administration of the drug to a secretary, she fell asleep for 24 h, developed low blood pressure, marked bradycardia, and dryness of the mouth. Clonidine was subsequently developed for its blood-lowering effect and introduced into the clinical routine in 1966.

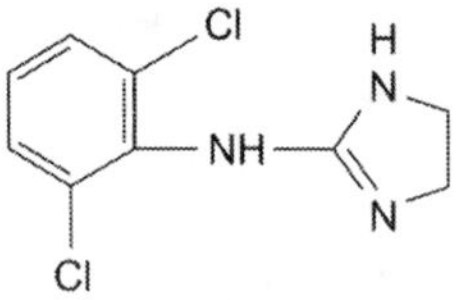

Clonidine

e. Lead Discovery Based on Use of Traditional Medicine or Natural Products

Quinine

The isolation of the anti-malarial drug quinine from the bark of cinchona trees (e.g. *Cinchona officinalis*) was accomplished by the French chemists Pierre-Joseph Pelletier and Joseph-Bienaimé Caventou in 1820. The bark had long been used by indigenous peoples for the treatment of fevers. Spanish Jesuit missionaries, after the conquest of the Inca Empire in Peru in the late sixteenth and early seventeenth century, learned of this use from the natives and found that the bark was effective in preventing and treating malaria. They brought this knowledge, along with the bark, back to Europe, where it became widely used and was often referred to as "Peruvian bark." With quinine as the model, chemists subsequently synthesized the antimalarial drugs chloroquine and mefloquine, and they have continued to modify the basic structure of quinine to produce even more effective agents, such as the new antimalarial drug, bulaquine (developed by CDRI).

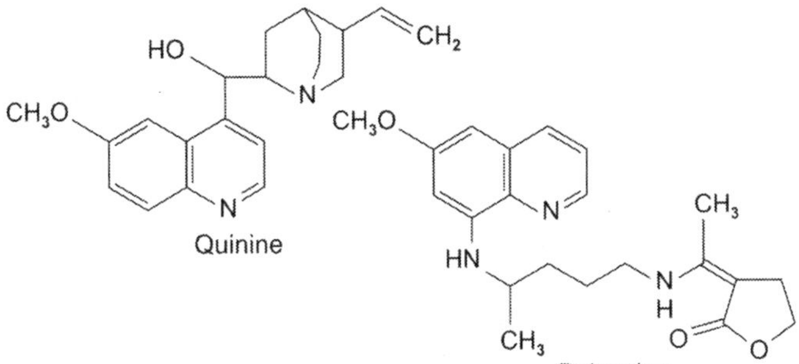

Quinine

Bulaquine

Artemisinin

The Sweet Wormwood plant (*Artemesia annua*) was also used as a treatment for fevers in China for more than 2,000 years (it is called *qing hao* in Chinese), but it was not until 1972 that the active compound artemisinin (*qing hao su*, which means the active principle of qing hao) was extracted and later identified as a potent anti malarial drug by Chinese scientists. This effort was part of a systematic examination at that time of indigenous plants in China as sources of new medicines. More soluble derivatives, artemether, artether, *etc.* have been developed in recent years to overcome its drawback.

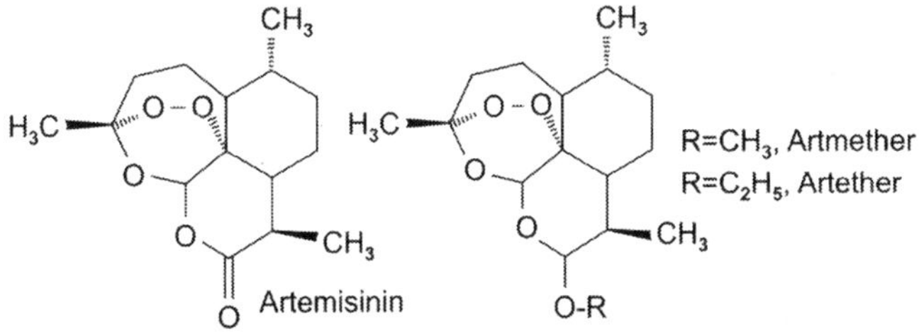

R=CH₃, Artmether
R=C₂H₅, Artether

Artemisinin

These medicines, in combination with other antimalarials such as mefloquine, have proved highly effective in treating malaria, particularly the most deadly form caused by *Plasmodium falciparum*, which has become increasingly resistant to the first-line treatments chloroquine and sulphadoxine-pyrimethamine—in Asia, South and Central America, and Africa.

Some examples of drugs from plants that served as models for the next generation of drugs are exemplified as follows: Khellin [from *Ammi visnaga* (L.) was used as a bronchodilator in the United States until it was shown to produce nausea and vomiting after prolonged use. In 1955, a group of chemists in England set about to synthesize Khellin analogs as potential bronchodilators with fewer side effects. This eventually led to the discovery of chromolyn (used as sodium cromoglycate), which stabilized cell membranes in the lungs to prevent the allergen induced release of the substance ultimately causing bronchoconstriction in allergic asthma patients. Further studies elsewhere led to the synthesis of amiodarone, a useful antiarrythmic agent.

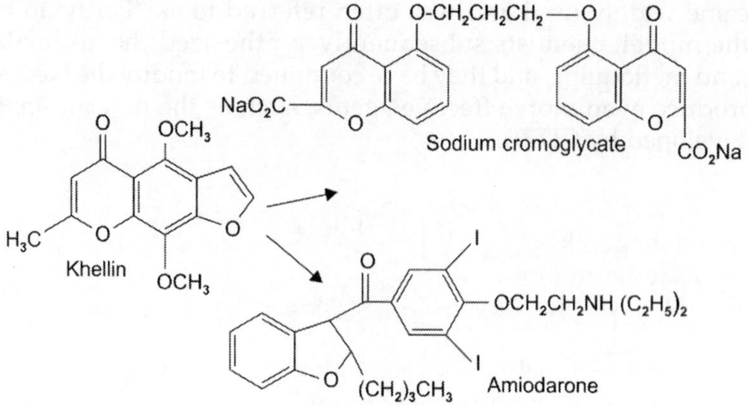

Papaverine, useful as a smooth muscle relaxant, provided the basic structure for verapamil, a drug used to treat hypertension.

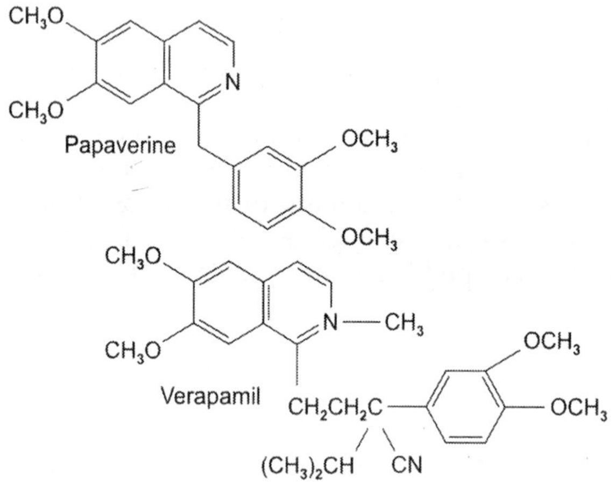

Galegine was isolated as an active antihyperglycemic agent from the plant *Galega officinalis* L. This plant was used ethnomedically for the treatment of diabetes. Galegine provided the template for the synthesis of metformin and opened up interest in the synthesis of other biguanidine-type anti diabetic drugs.

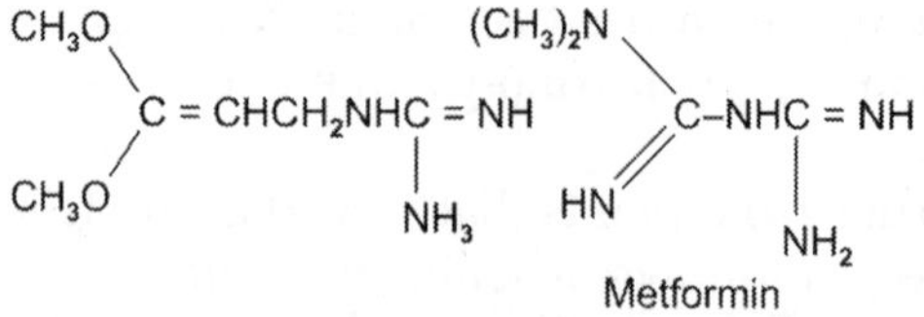

Epibatidine is a potent analgesic isolated from the skin of *Epipedobates tricolor* (phantasmal poison frog). Epibatidine is several hundred times stronger than morphine. However, the therapeutic dose of the compound is close to the toxic dose, driving the development of synthetic analogues. Epibatidine serves as a lead compound for potential novel analgesics. To date, synthetic analogues have not reached clinical use.

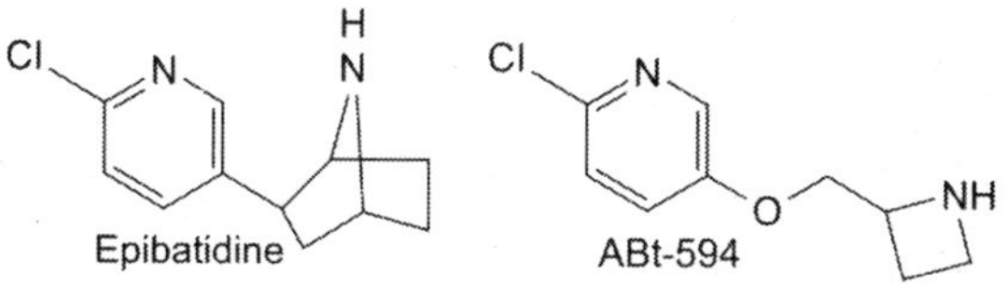

Epibatidine

ABt-594
Failed phase (clinical trial II)

Teprotide is a nonapeptide isolated from the venom of *Bothrops jararaca* (Brazilian pit viper). It is a known inhibitor of the Angiotensin Converting Enzyme (ACE). Teprotide was used as a lead compound for the development of the ACE inhibitor, captopril.

From January 1981 to June 2006, 1,184 new drugs and drug candidates were reported. Approximately 70% of these compounds were either natural products, derived from natural products, or inspired by natural products. Examples of natural products and respective synthetic drugs they have inspired include ephedrine and propranolol (Inderal), HMG-CoA and rosuvastatin (Rusvas) and 2'-deoxyguanosine and acyclovir (Zovir).

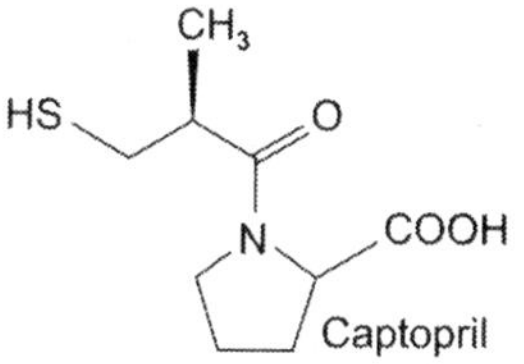

Captopril

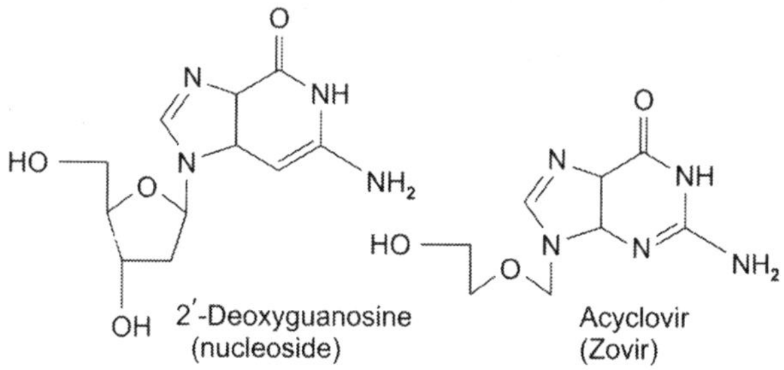

2'-Deoxyguanosine
(nucleoside)

Acyclovir
(Zovir)

f. Rational Approaches to Lead Discovery

Although serendipity played a important role in the pharmaceutical industry over the years, current drug discovery is an extraordinarily complicated, expensive and time-consuming process, with strategies involving screening natural products, mimicking biological substrates (and metabolites), and the use of structure-based drug design. Drug design, often referred to as rational drug design or simply rational design, is the inventive process of finding new medications based on the knowledge of a biological target. Generally, the rational development of a new drug follows a three-step process. Step I: Initially, a target, such as a receptor or enzyme, has to be identified relating to a particular disease state. Step II: This target then has to be fully characterized (structurally and functionally) and, StepIII: finally, a molecule must be designed that binds to it. The knowledge about the receptors and their mode of interaction with drug molecules plays an important role in drug design. The knowledge may be used to develop the conformationally bioactive skeleton having three dimensional complementary to a receptor. Greater potency, higher selectivity and less adverse effects are expected by reducing the flexibility of the drug structure. For example, replacement of terminal N, N-diethyl amino group by piperidine to make it good access of basic group at the anionic site of receptor led to development of major tranquilizer, local anesthetic, antihistaminic, spasmolytic drugs.

Secondly, most of the diseases develop from the imbalance of endogenous substances.

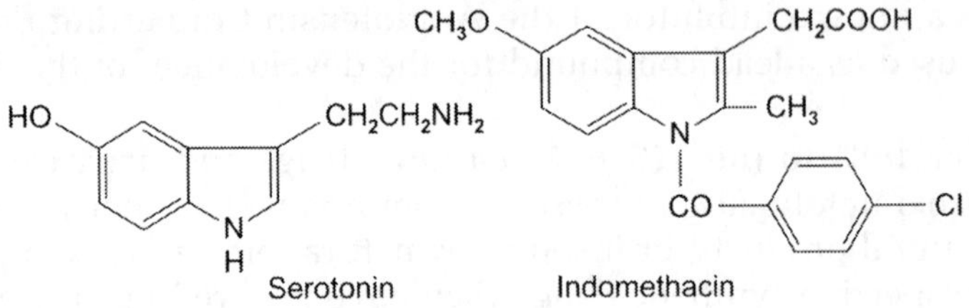

Serotonin   Indomethacin

The imbalance may be corrected by agonism or antagonism of the receptor. For example, it was thought that serotonin is a possible mediator of inflammation. By considering the skeleton of serotonin as pharmacophore, anti-inflammatory drug, indomethacin was developed.

The discovery of cimetidine (Tagamet) starts with a validated biological target and ends up with a drug that optimally interacts with the target and triggers the desired biological action. Histamine triggers release of stomach acid. Hence, there is need of histamine antagonist to prevent stomach acid release by histamine. It is a **validated biological target**.

Histamine   Histamine analogs

N-Guanyl histamine

Cimetidine   N-C≡N

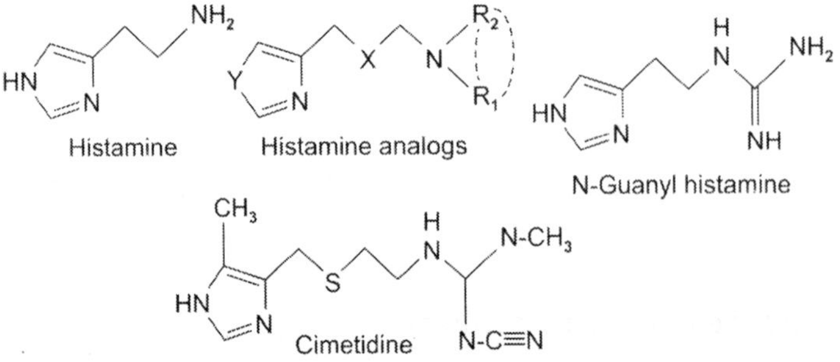

Histamine analogs were synthesized with systematically varied structures (chemical modification), and Screened. N-guanyl-histamine showed some antagonist properties = Lead compound. Replacement with appropriate group led to an effective and well-tolerated product-cimetidine.

Selective serotonin reuptake inhibitors (SSRIs), a class of antidepressants were also developed using rational drug design. These are used for treating depression, anxiety disorders and some personality disorders. These drugs are designed to allow the available neurotransmitter serotonin to be utilized more efficiently. A low level of utilization of serotonin is currently seen as one among several neurochemical symptoms of depression. Low levels of serotonin in turn can be caused by an anxiety disorder because serotonin is needed to metabolize stress hormones. These medications evolve their effects at the serotonin transporter. They increase the extracellular level of the neurotransmitter serotonin by inhibiting its reuptake into the presynaptic cell. They have no or only weak effects on other monoamine transporters, thus having little direct influence on the level of other neurotransmitters

Some of the most ambitious efforts using rational drug design approach so far have involved HIV. Several potent inhibitors of HIV protease, an enzyme that is essential for the viral life cycle, were designed specifically to jam the structure of this protease; some are now undergoing clinical trials. However, HIV mutates so rapidly that it is probably the most difficult of all targets for drugs. Using this approach, hepatic hydroxyl methyl glutaryl coenzyme A (HMGA) reductase inhibitors and angiotensin-converting enzyme (ACE) inhibitors used for the treatment of hypertension were developed.

Optimization of Lead Structure

Once the lead structure is identified, it is easy to exploit. For example, cocaine is a lead compound which is optimized to develop the improvised lead compound. From the improvised lead compound, benzocaine, procaine and procainamide are designed.

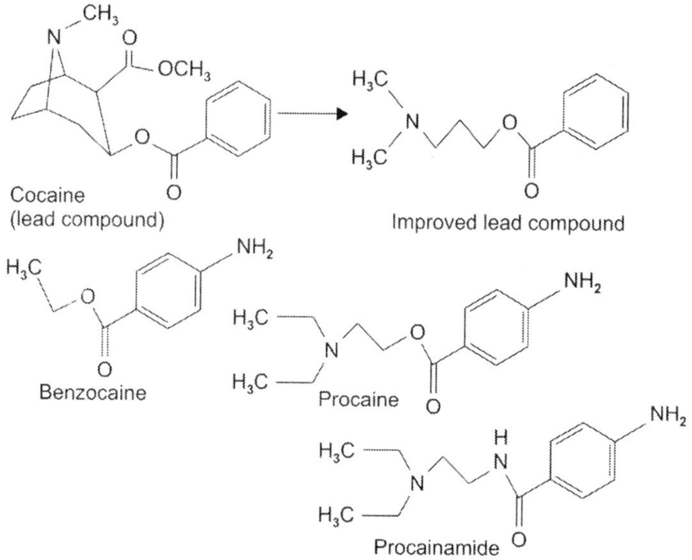

Cocaine
(lead compound)

Improved lead compound

Benzocaine

Procaine

Procainamide

Various approaches are employed in order to improve the desired pharmacological properties of lead nucleus. Some of them are as follows:

a. Identification of Pharmacophore

Almost every molecule consists of both essential and nonessential parts. Essential part is important for drug-receptor interaction (pharmacodynamic activity) and non-essential part affects the pharmacokinetic features.

The concerning groups in the molecule that interact with receptor are known as *bioactive functional groups*. The nature of such bioactive functional groups along with inter atomic distances is known as, *Pharmacophore*. Once such pharmacophore is identified, structural modification can be done to improve pharmacokinetic properties of a drug. For example, morphine is a prototype narcotic agent. Several derivatives of morphine like pentazocine, levalorphan, *etc.* are synthesized and from that it was

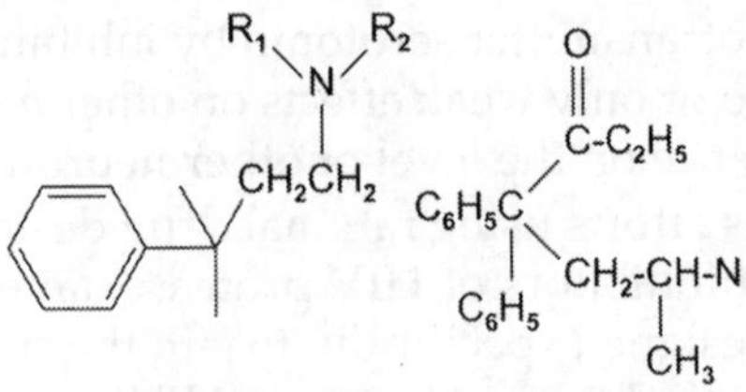

Pharmacophore   Methadone
for narcotic drug

concluded that presence of phenyl ring, asymmetric carbon atom, ethylenic bridge and tertiary nitrogen are found to be minimum requirement for a narcotic analgesic action.

Hence, pharmacophore of morphine has been recognized and was used to get equipotent analgesic drug, methadone with less addictive properties.

Similarly, aspirin and its analogs were developed by considering salicylic acid as an active lead compound. Earlier, salicylic acid was reported to be present in the plant, *Salix alba* as glucoside, Salicin. This plant was used for the treatment of rheumatic disorder.

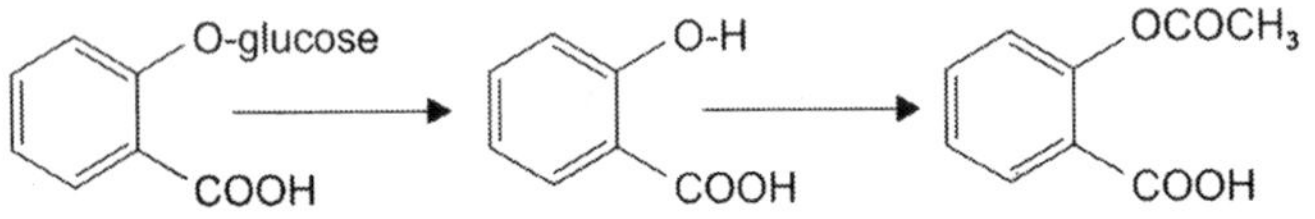

Salicin   Salicylic acid   Aspirin

b. Functional Group Optimization

The activity of a drug can be correlated to its structure in term of the contribution of its functional group to the lipophilicity, electronic and steric features of the drug nucleus. Hence, by selecting appropriate functional group, one can decide the distribution pattern and can avoid the occurrence of side effects. For example, the amino group of carbutamide (antibacterial agent) was replaced by a methyl group to give tolbutamide (antidiabetic drug).

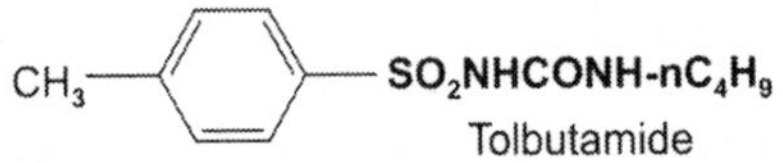

Tolbutamide

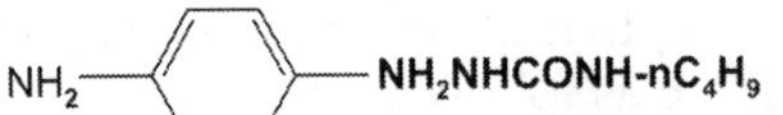

Carbutamide

Similarly, removal of sulphonamide side chain of chlorothiazide (an antihypertensive with diuretic activity) helped to design the diazoxide (an antihypertensive drug without diuretic activity)

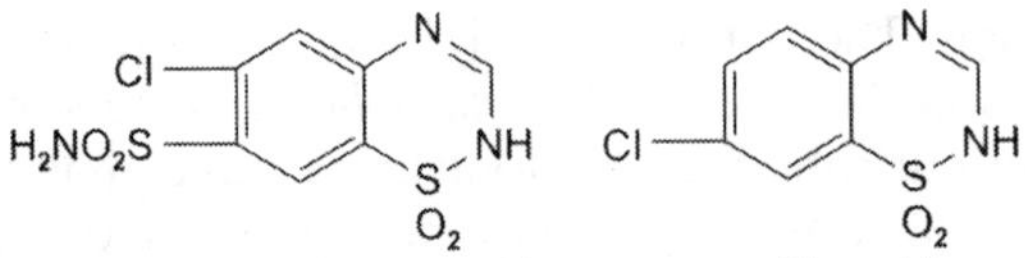

Chlorothiazide   Diazoxide

c. Structure–Activity Relationship (SAR) Studies

SAR studies involve the interpretation of activity in terms of structural features of a drug molecule. A generalized conclusion can be made after knowing the biological activity of sufficient number of analogues. For example, sulphonamides are found to be associated with diuretic and antidiabetic activities in addition to their antibacterial activity. The generalized structures required for individual activity are represented in Fig. 2.1.

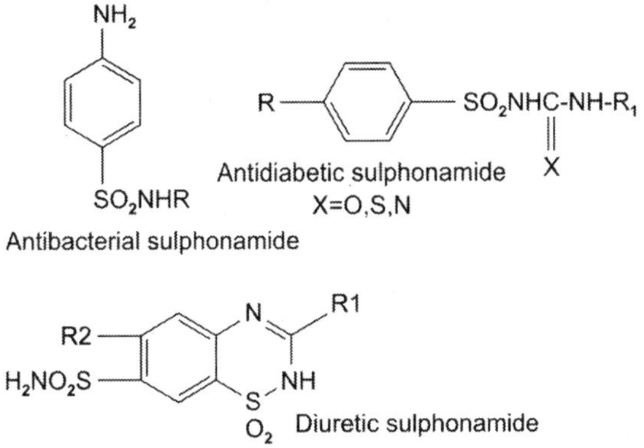

Fig. 2.1: Generalized structure for various activities in sulphonamides

d. Homologation

The homologous series is a group of compounds that differ by a constant unit, generally CH_2 group. Usually increasing the length of saturated carbon side chain from one (CH_3) to 5(pentyl) to 9(nonyl) increases the pharmacological activity. Further increase in carbon atom chain results in decrease in activity. This is due to increase in lipophilicity beyond optimum value. For example, 4-alkyl substituted resorcinol derivatives are used as topical anesthetics in throat lozenges but it shows maximum activity when it is substituted with hexyl group. Similarly, maximum hypnotic activity is obtained from 1-hexanol to 1-octanol.

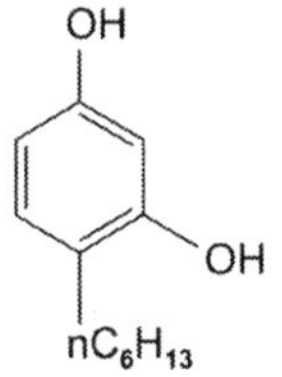

n-Hexyl resorcinol

Homologation of the N-alkyl chain in norapomorphine from methyl $(R=CH_3)$ to ethyl $(R=C_2H_5)$ to propyl $(R=C_3H_7)$ increases the emetic response in dogs and

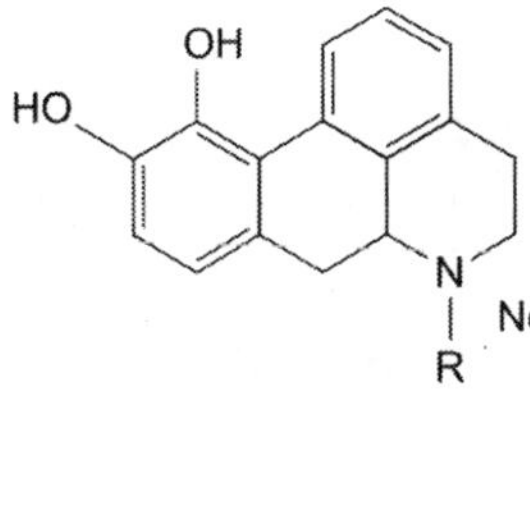

Norapomorphine, R=H

stereotype response in rodents. The homolog, *n*-butyl(R= *n*-C₄H₉) demonstrated a tremendous loss in potency and activity compared to lower homologs.

e. Cyclization of the Side Chain

Change in potency or change in activity can be brought out by transformation of alkyl chain into cyclic analogs. For example, chlorpromazine (i) has more neuroleptic activity than its cyclic analog (ii).

Similarly, the compound (iii) has antidepressant activity than neuroleptic activity while in compound (iv), the antiemetic activity is greatly enhanced.

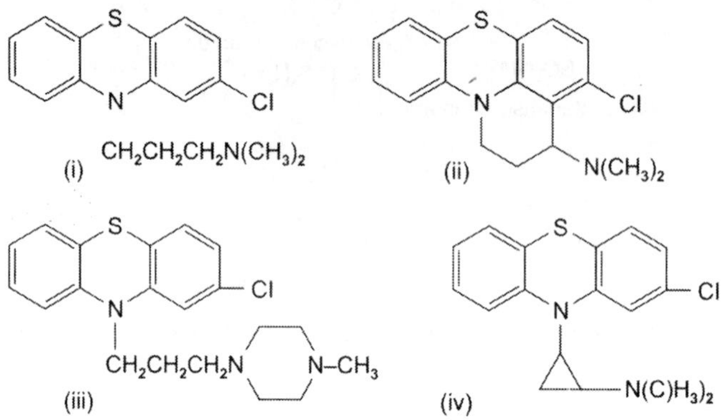

The local anesthetic drug, Bupivacaine has arisen from a modification of side chain.

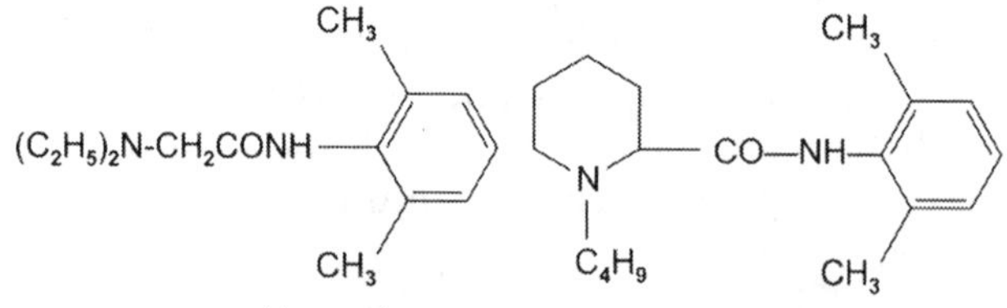

Lignocaine   Bupivacaine

f. Reversal of Functional Groups

The reversal of the peptide functional groups is often used in peptide chemistry. The retropeptides obtained are generally more resistant to enzymatic attacks. The same strategy is applied to non peptide compounds. The example of this is development of neo-orthoform (orthocaine) from orthoform by reversal of group.

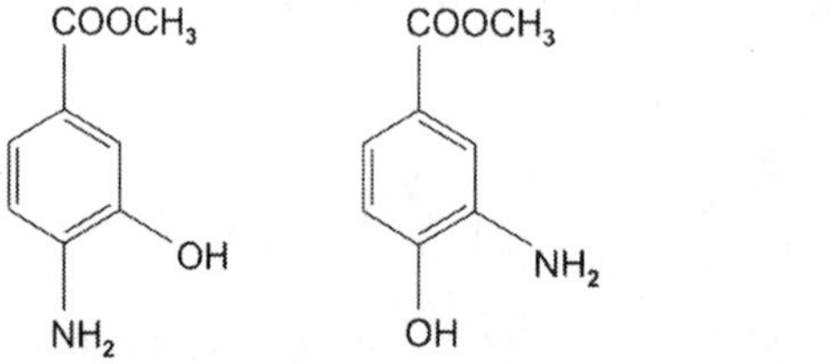

Orthoform   Neo-orthoform (Orthocaine)

The unwanted side effects, often associated with *p*-aromatic compounds (para effects) are abolished in *m*-amino isomer whereas the local anesthetic activity is retained.

The inversion of the ester functional group of meperidine leads to 1-methyl-4-phenyl-4-propionoxy piperidine which is five times more potent as an analgesic drug than meperidine.

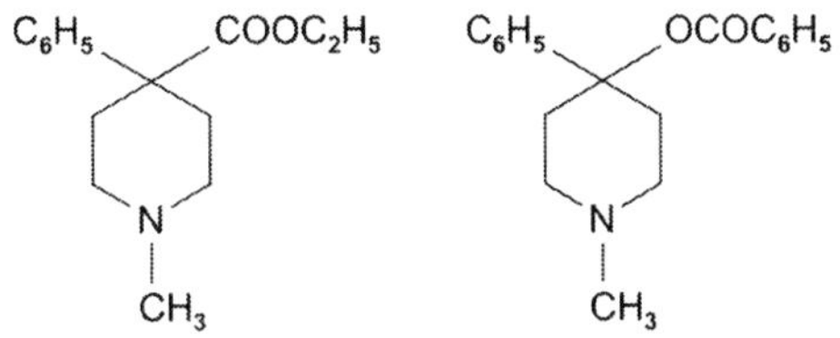

Meperidine   Inverted ester

Similarly, the NSAIDs, clometacin and indomethacin has same functional groups but at inverse position.

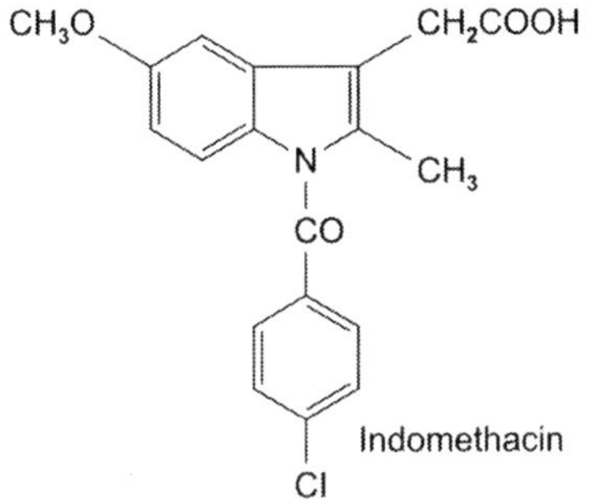

Indomethacin 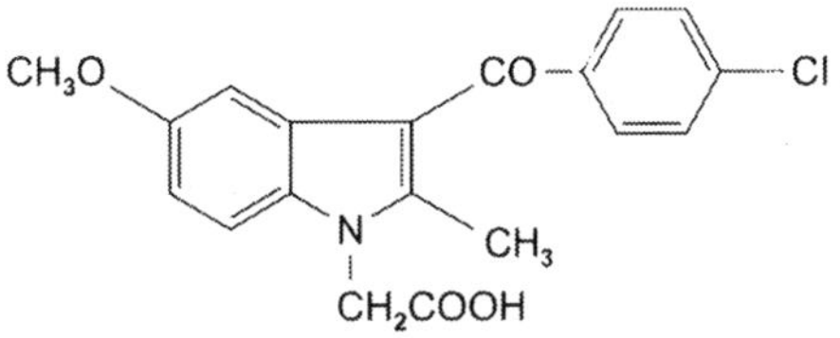   Clometacin

g. Bioisosterism

The aim of molecular modification is usually to improve potency, selectivity, duration of action and reduce toxicity. Most of this work is based on the phenomenon of bioisosterism. It is discussed in Chapter 3.

h. Computer-Aided Drug Design

Traditional drug design is an expensive and laborious process of developing new or better medicine. This process has its origin in herbal remedies dating back millennia. Only since the last century drugs had a (semi)synthetic origin. The first hit compounds often lack both potency and safety, and must therefore be optimized. Historically, this was a trial-and-error process for developing rational strategies to improve potency. As with any data handling procedures, computers have also become a more prominent and ubiquitous tool in drug discovery since the 1980s. The crossover between computational and pharmaceutical research is typically designated as computer-aided drug design (CADD) (Fig. 2.2).

The main purpose of CADD is to speed up and rationalize the drug design process while reducing costs. The aim of the earliest phase in computer aided drug discovery is to identify the first hit compounds, which is sometimes attempted by high-throughput screening (HTS), the testing of many thousands of compounds with a suitable activity assay. The *in silico* counterpart of *in vitro* HTS is referred to as virtual screening and aims at filtering libraries of molecules using computational methods to prioritize those most likely to be active for a given target. Later in the drug discovery pipeline the potency of the hit and lead compounds needs to be improved. New derivatives are designed with or without a different scaffold at the core of the molecule.

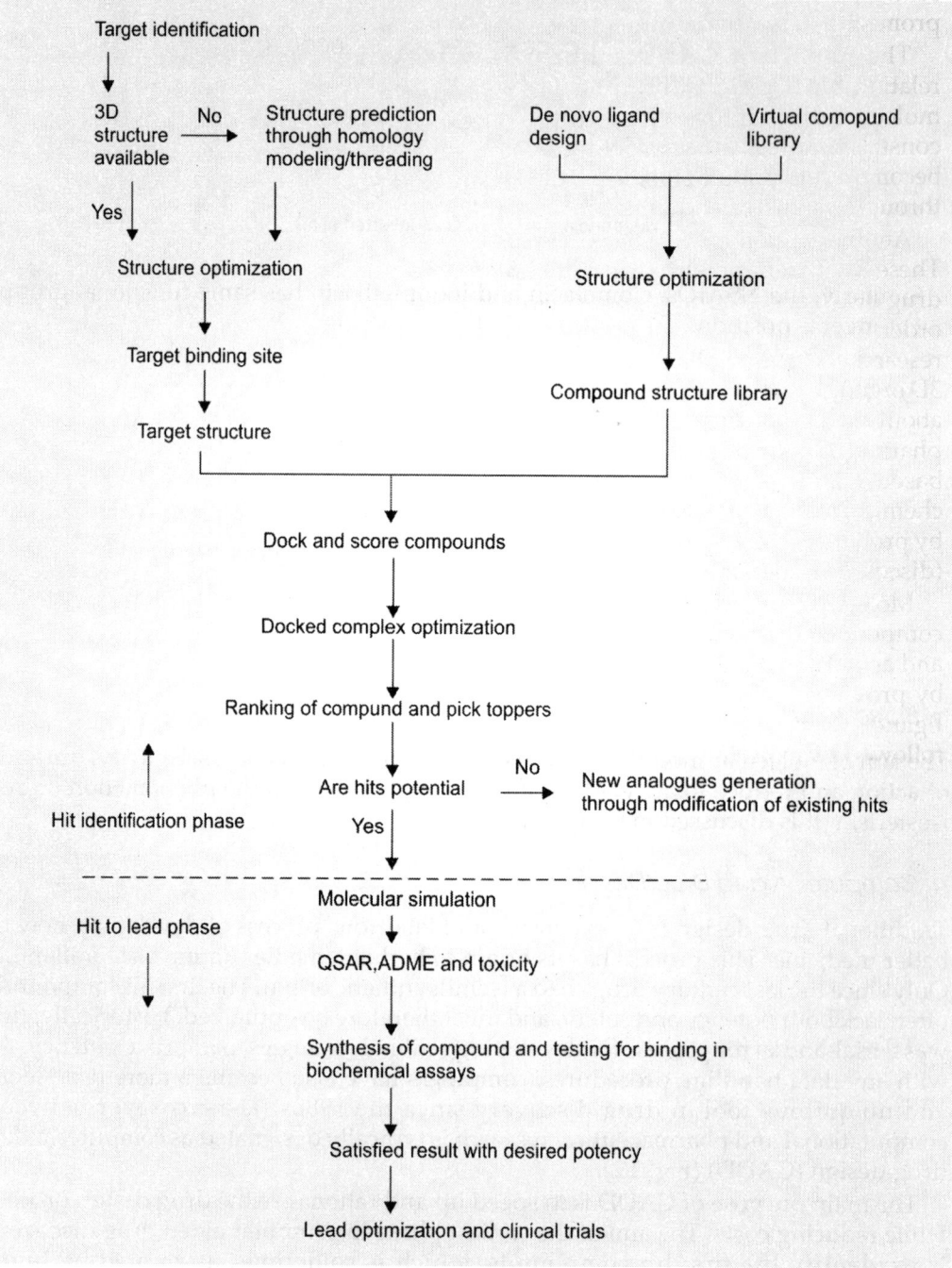

Fig. 2.2: Role of CADD in drug discovery

The ultimate goal is to design highly potent and specific molecules which also have a suitable intellectual property position. This can be achieved by classical medicinal chemistry approaches, where the design can be based on the observed structure–activity relationships (SAR) or based on structural information. Computational methods however can also be used to create diverse derivatives based on different scaffolds, and then score them for improved potency. This prioritizes the most promising derivatives from a very wide chemical space in a relatively short time.

The important CADD subfield is quantitative structure activity/property relationship (QSAR/QSPR), in which the physicochemical properties (as calculated by molecular descriptors) of a set of inhibitors are related to the biological activity to construct a predictive model for novel compound (to be used as drug). QSAR has become a very popular tool to profile novel inhibitors accurately in silico without going through expensive and time-consuming in vitro and in vivo assays.

Another option for CADD is 3D-pharmacophore modeling and molecular docking. These are two basic virtual screening techniques that may play an important role in drug discovery. Pharmacophore modeling is most often applied to virtual screening in order to identify molecules triggering the desired biological effect. For this purpose, researchers create a pharmacophore model (query) that most likely encodes the correct 3D organization of the required interaction pattern. Depending on how much is known about the particular protein target, different options are available to construct such a pharmacophoric model. A pharmacophore model can be established either in a ligand based manner, by superposing a set of active molecules and extracting common chemical features that are essential for their bioactivity, or in a structure-based manner, by probing possible interaction points between the macromolecular target and ligands (discussed in detail in Chapter 7).

Molecular docking is a method which predicts the binding orientation of candidate compounds to their protein targets (receptor) in order to in turn evaluate the affinity and activity of the ligands. It is always utilized for screening the initial results further by providing more structural information and the pattern of receptor recognizing ligands. Once lead compound is identified, it is optimized and then synthesized followed by experimental trials.

3 | Bioisosterism—A Useful Strategy for Drug Development

INTRODUCTION

Bioisosterism has unique importance in the field of pharmaceutical sciences and is applied to curtail side effects or to alter the biological activity of a lead molecule. In the biomedical field, the aim of exchanging one bioisostere for another is to boost the preferred pharmacological, biological or physical qualities of a substance without making substantial changes in the chemical skeleton (for example to change bioavailability, reduce toxicity or modify the activity of the lead compound).

Isostere

The isostere concept was formulated by **Irving Langmuir** in 1919. The octet theory of valence indicates that if compounds having the same number of atoms, have also the same total number of electrons, the electrons may arrange themselves in the same manner. In this case, the compounds or groups of atoms are said to be isosteric. Hence, isosteres were initially defined as those compounds or groups of atoms that have the same number and arrangement of electrons.

Such compounds should show remarkable similarity in physical properties, that is, in those properties which do not involve a separation of the atoms in the molecule.

Bioisostere

The term "bioisostere" was introduced by **Harris Friedman** in 1950. Bioisosteres are atoms or group of molecules that fit the broadest definition for isosteres. They are similar in chemical and physical properties, thus producing broadly similar biological properties. The extensive application of isosterism to modify a part of a biologically active molecule to get another one of similar activity, has given rise to the term of **bioisosterism**. Many heterocycles, when appropriately substituted exhibits bioisosterism. It represents an approach used by the medicinal chemist for the rational modification of lead compounds into safer and more clinically effective agents. In drug design, the purpose of exchanging one bioisostere for another is for the following reasons:

1. To enhance the desired biological or physical properties of a compound without making significant changes in chemical structure.
2. To attenuate toxicity.
3. To modify the activity of the lead compound.
4. To alter the metabolism of the lead.

Due to molecular modification and substitution, a little change in activity (i.e. either increase or decrease in affinity or efficacy) can occur but other parameters are generally not changed like:

    i. Size

    ii. Shape (bond angles and hybridization)

    iii. Electronic distribution (polarizability, inductive effects, charge, dipoles)

    iv. Lipid solubility

    v. Water solubility

    vi. pKa

    vii. Chemical reactivity (including likelihood of metabolism)

    viii. Hydrogen bonding capacity (important for target binding), *etc.*

CLASSIFICATION OF BIOISOSTERES

In 1970, Burger classified and subdivided bioisosteres into two broad categories according to the degree of electronic and steric factors.

A. Classic Isosteres

They obey steric and electronic definition. These are further classified into:

1. Univalent atoms and groups
   a. CH_3, NH_2, OH, F, Cl (for example the replacement of H by F atom in uracil. Since, steric parameters of H and F atoms are similar).
   b. Cl, PH_2, SH
   c. Br, i-Pr
   d. I, t-Bu
2. Bivalent atoms and groups
   a. $-CH_2$, -NH-,-O-,-S-, -Se-
   b. $-COCH_2R$,-CONHR, $-CO_2R$,-COSR
3. Trivalent atoms and groups
   a. –CH=. –N=
   b. –P=,-As=
4. Tetravalent atoms

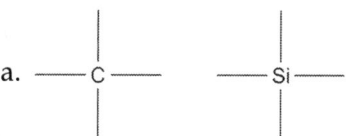

    b. =C=, $=N^+=$, $=P^+=$

5. Ring equivalents
   a. –CH=CH-,-S- (e.g. benzene, thiophene)
   b. –CH=,-N= (e.g. benzene, pyridine)
   c. –O-,-S-,-CH_2-,-NH- (e.g. tetrahydrofuran, tetrahydrothiophene, cyclopentane, pyrolidine)

B. Nonclassic bioisosteres

- They do not obey the steric and electronic definition of classical isosteres.
- They do not have the same number of atoms as the substituent or moiety for which they are used as a replacement (Table 3.1).

Table 3.1: Nonclassic bioisosters

1. Carbonyl group

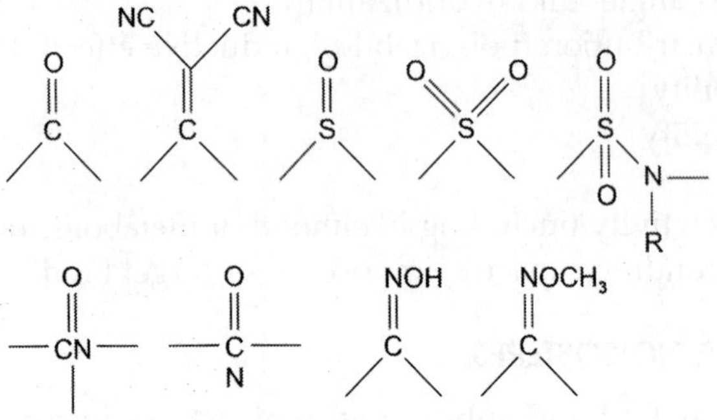

2. Carboxylic acid group

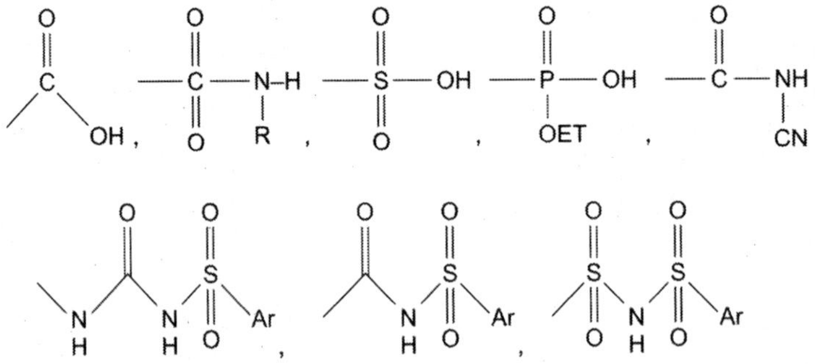

3. Amide group

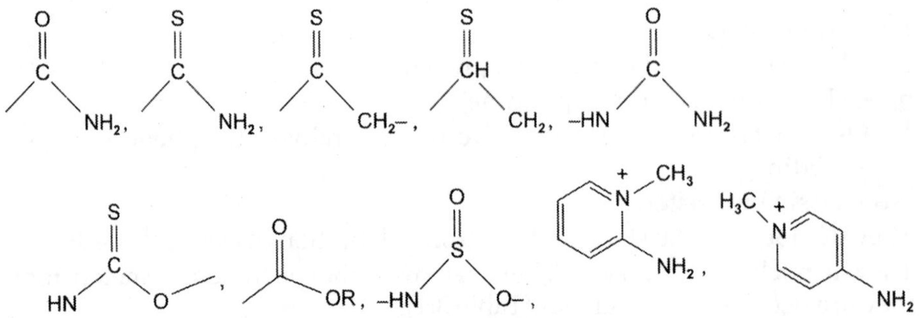

4. Ester group

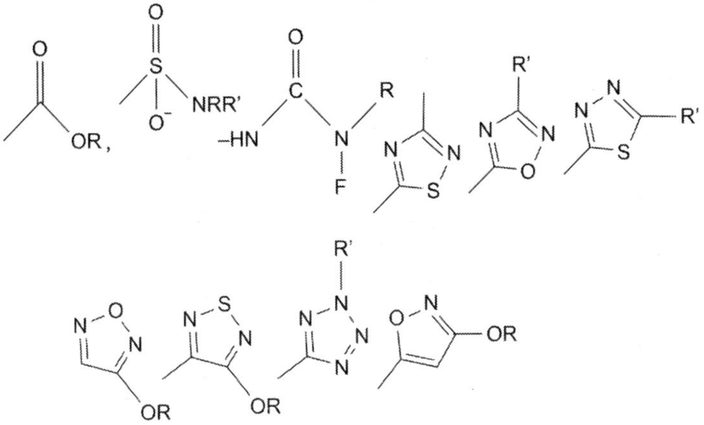

5. Hydroxyl group

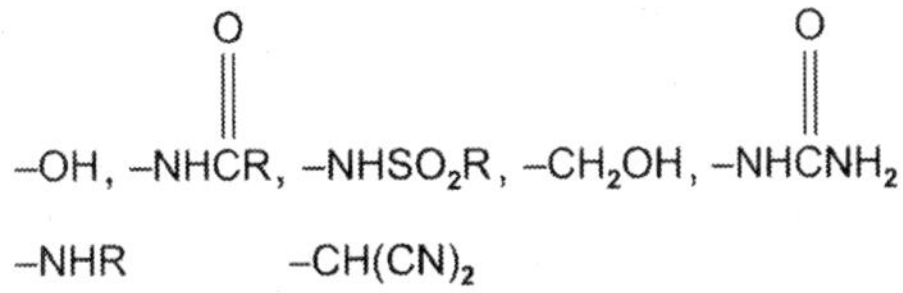

$$-OH, \quad -NH\overset{O}{\overset{\|}{C}}R, \quad -NHSO_2R, \quad -CH_2OH, \quad -NH\overset{O}{\overset{\|}{C}}NH_2$$

$$-NHR \qquad -CH(CN)_2$$

6. Catechol

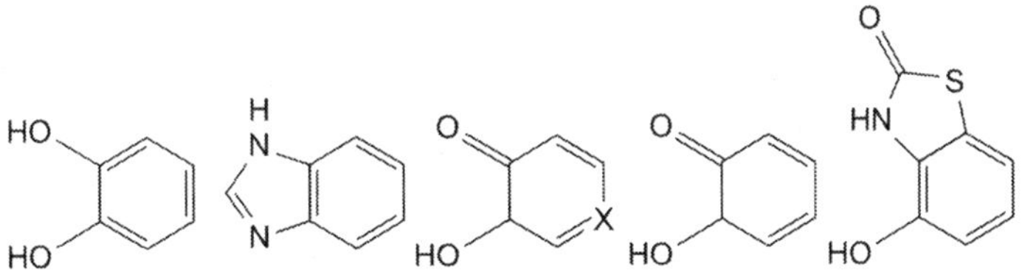

X=O, NR

7. Halogen

$$X \qquad CF_3 \qquad CN \qquad N(CN)_2 \qquad C(CN)_3$$

8. Thioether

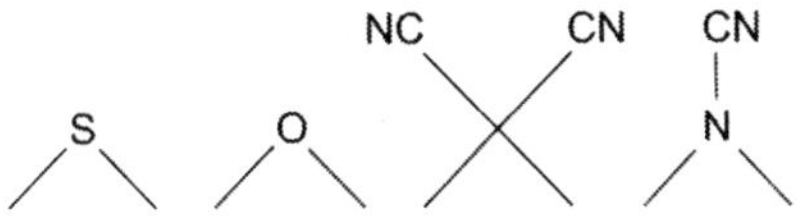

9. Thiourea

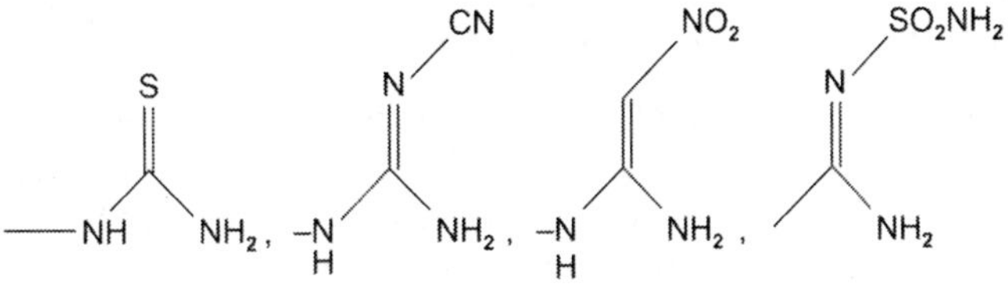

10. Azomethine

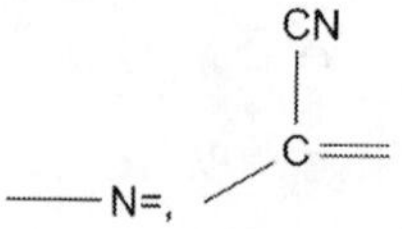

— N=, and a C group with CN substituent and triple bond

11. Pyridine

NO₂   R   +NR₃

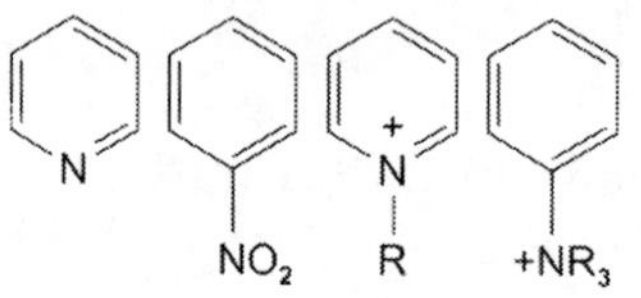

12. Benzene

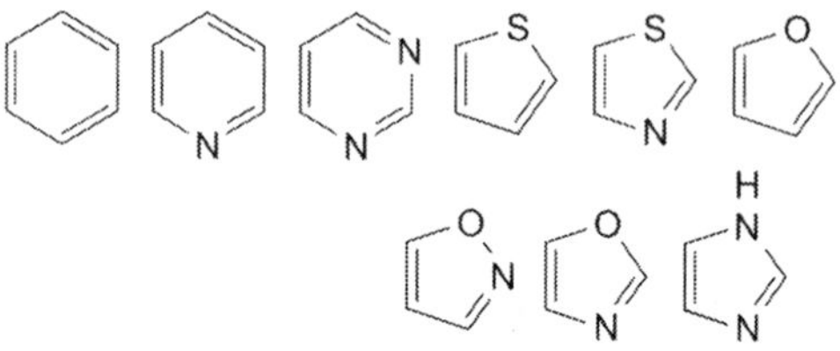

13. Ring equivalent

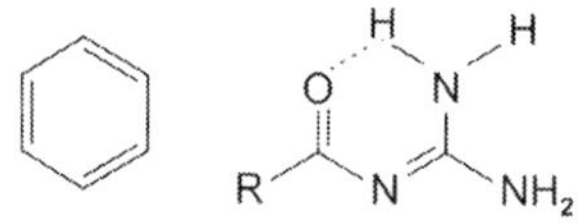

14. Spacer group

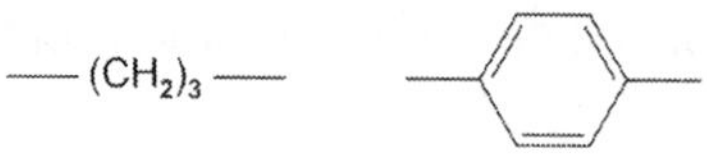

— (CH₂)₃ —

15. Hydrogen

H F

16. Carboxylic acid isosteres: The COOH isoster is present in Angiotensin-II receptor antagonists. These antagonists provide instructive insight to carboxylic acid isoster design, since binding affinity to receptors in a series of biphenyl acid is quite sensitive to the identity of the acidic element.

17. Phenyl ring isosteres: The phenyl ring can often be replaced by a heteroaromatic ring or a saturated ring. For example: Cyclopropane as phenyl isoster. It was explained as mimetic of phenyl ring in an effort to identify compound with decreased molecular weight and lower lipophilicity.

Applications of Bioisosterism in Drug Design

Monovalent Atoms and Group

i. The bioisosteric modification of oral hypoglycemic drug, carbutamide by replacing the –NH$_2$ with chlorine and CH$_3$ group gave chlorpropamide and tolbutamide respectively. Both of these have extended biological half lives and reduced toxicity (Table 3.2).

Table 3.2: Half life of oral hypoglycemic sulfonylurea drugs

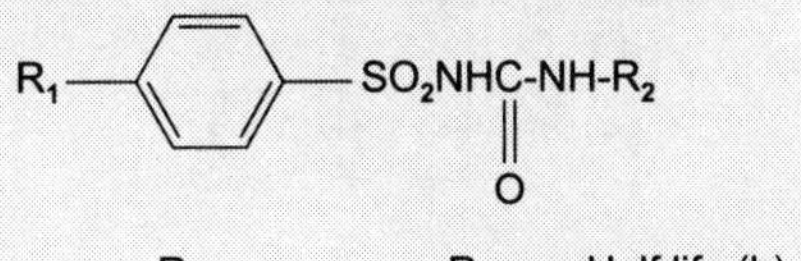

$$R_1 - \underset{}{\bigcirc} - SO_2NHC-NH-R_2$$
$$\underset{O}{\|}$$

Drug	R_1	R_2	Half life (h)
Carbutamide	-NH$_2$	-nC$_4$H$_9$	3
Tolbutamide	-CH$_3$	-$\underline{n}$C$_4$H$_9$	5.7
Chlorpropamide	-Cl	-nC$_3$H$_7$	33

ii. The substitution of hydrogen atom by fluorine is a good example of isosteric replacement to develop antineoplastic drug, 5-flurouracil. Steric parameters for hydrogen and fluorine are similar; their van der Wall's radii being 1.2 and 1.35Å respectively.

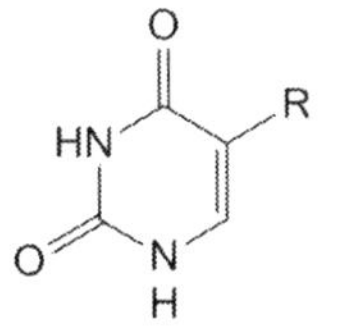

Uracil, R=H
5-Fluorouracil, R=F

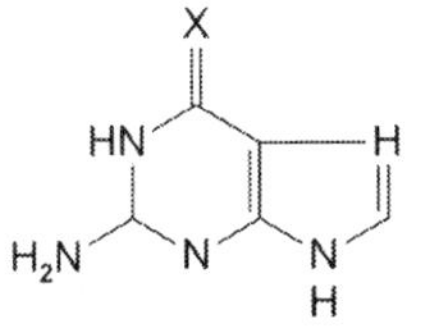

Guanine, X=O
Thioguanine, X=S

iv. 6-Thioguanine is a purine antimetabolite, developed by isosteric replacement of hydroxyl group by thio group.

v. Zidovudine (AZT), an important chemotherapeutic agent available for the treatment of acquired human immunodeficiency syndrome, was discovered from the properties identified in nucleosides isolated from seaweed. The structural analysis of AZT, a powerful inhibitor of transcriptase reverse enzyme, enables us to ascertain the existence of a classic bioisosteric relationship of monovalent groups between the nucleoside thymidine (endogenous substrate for the synthesis of DNA and RNA) and AZT, exemplified by the presence of the hydroxyl (OH) unit in nucleoside and azido (N$_3$) group present in AZT. Furthermore, although these are classic monovalent isosteres but the OH and N$_3$ groups possess dramatic electronic differences, easily demonstrated by simple functional analysis.

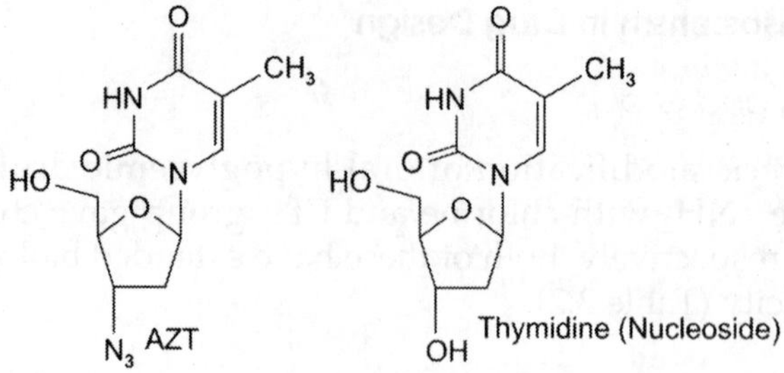

AZT

Thymidine (Nucleoside)

vi. Examples of biosteric analogs in anti-inflammatory drugs

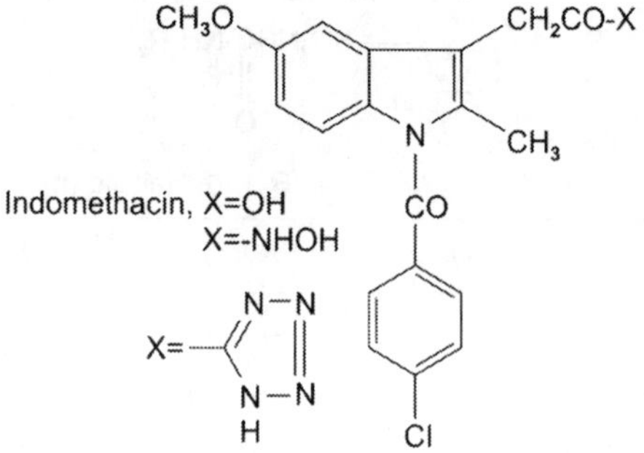

Indomethacin, X=OH
X=-NHOH

vii. The phenomenon of bioisosterism is also observed in antihistaminic drugs.

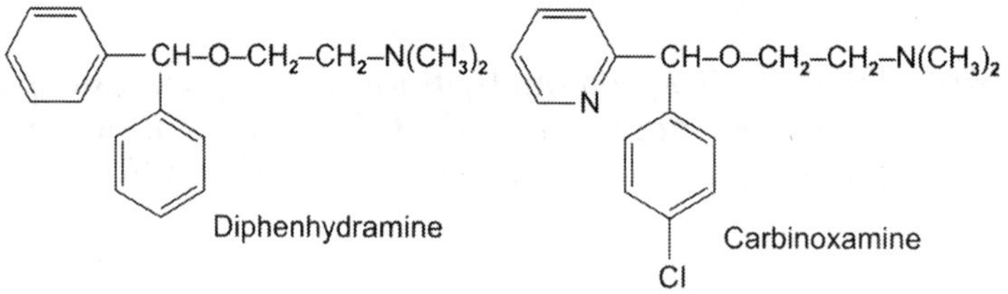

Diphenhydramine

Carbinoxamine

Carbinoxamine and diphenhydramine are similar in structure except in carbinoxamine, chlorine atom replaces the hydrogen atom. Both hydrogen and chlorine atoms are monovalent.

viii. Interchange of hydroxyl and amino groups: The best known example of classical isosteric substitution of an amino group for a hydroxyl group is illustrated by aminopterin (b) wherein the hydroxyl substituent of folic acid (a) has been substituted by an amino group. This represents a monovalent bioisosteric substitution at a carbon atom adjacent to a heterocyclic nitrogen atom.

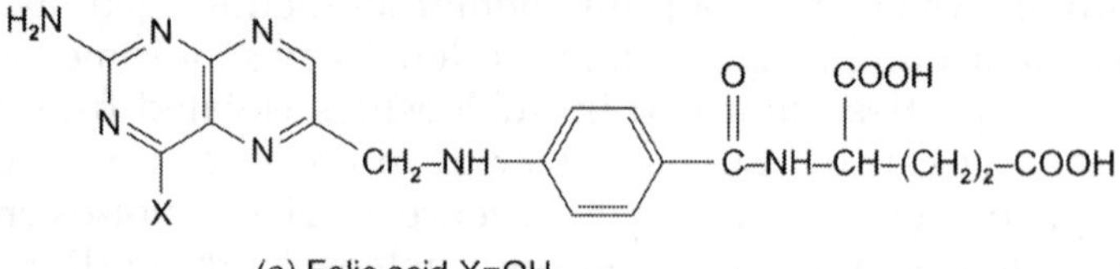

(a) Folic acid X=OH
(b) Aminopterin X=NH$_2$

ix. Replacement of chlorine with methyl group: The chlorine atom is often viewed to be isosteric and isolipophilic with the methyl group it is very often selected as a bioisosteric replacement because of its ability to alter the metabolism.

Replacement of a chloro atom (a) with a methyl substituent (b) can facilitate metabolism of a xenobiotic. Lipid-soluble chemicals tend to be distributed into adipose tissue where, unless they are metabolized, they tend to accumulate for long periods of time, e.g. DDT. The replacement of the trichloromethyl moiety with a tert-butyl group results in diminished persistence of this pesticide. The methyl substituent provides a site which is susceptible to metabolic degradation.

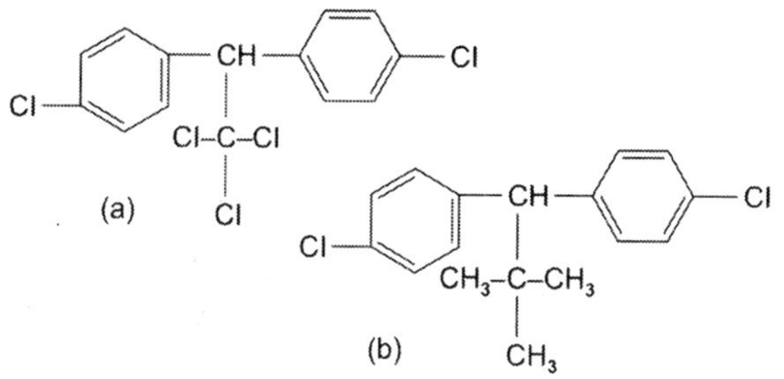

Divalent Replacements Involving Double Bonds

This subclass includes replacements of groups such as C=S, C=O, C=NH and C=C. The replacement of C=S with C=O in Tolrestat (a) an aldose reductase inhibitor, currently under study in human subjects for the treatment of diabetic neuropathy, resulted in oxo-tolrestat (b) which retained activity both *in vitro* and *in vivo* (Table 3.3).

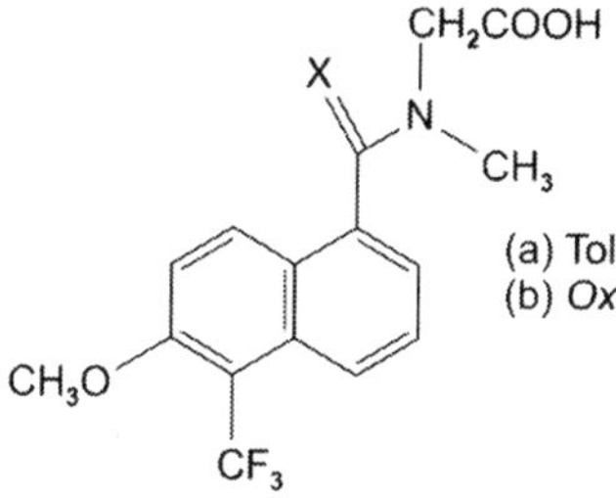

(a) Tolrestat, X=S
(b) Oxo-tolrestat, X=O

Table 3.3: Aldose reductase inhibitory activity of tolrestat and *oxo*-tolrestat

Compound	X	Aldose reductase inhibition	
		In vitro	*In vivo*
a	S	94	53
b	O	86	56

The bio-isosteric modification in procaine (local anesthetic drug) results in the development of Procainamide (antiarryhthmic drug) with change in activity. In this, divalent oxygen is replaced by –NH moiety.

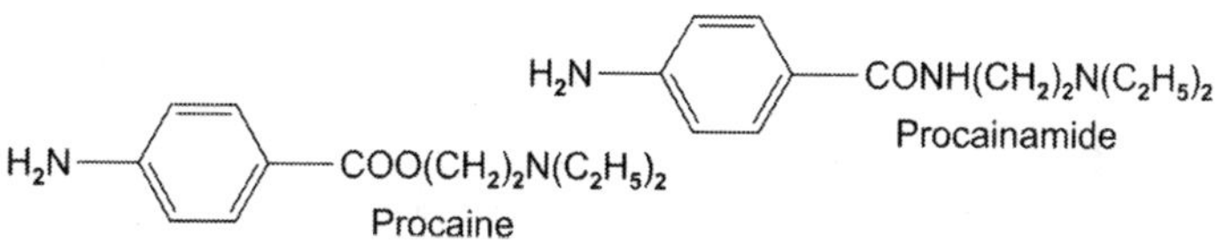

Bioisosteric replacement of carbonyl oxygen in hypoxanthine by S gives 6-mercaptopurine, a potent anticancer antimetabolite.

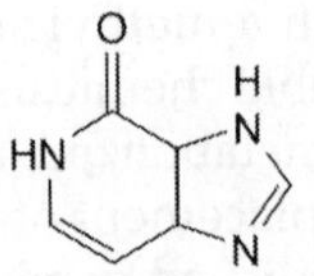

Hypoxanthine 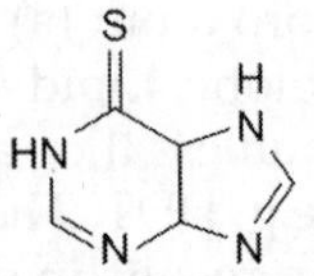   6-Mercaptopurine

The bioisosteric replacement of oxygen by sulphur in chlorpromazine gives oxygen isostere. This compound has 1/10 the soporific activity of the parent molecule.

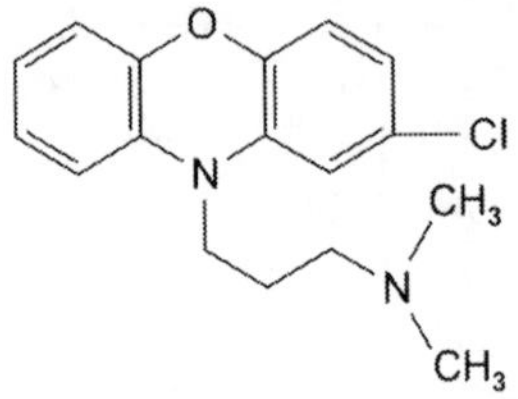

Oxygen biostere of chlorpromazine 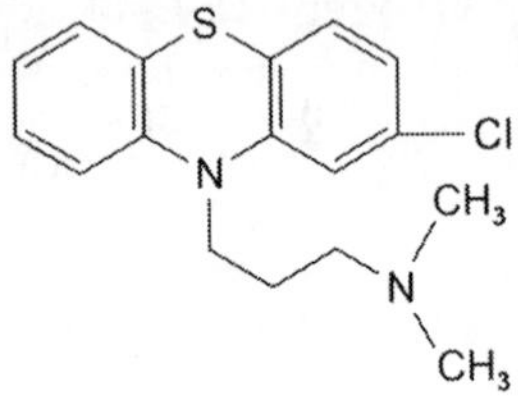   Chlorpromazine

Trivalent Atoms and Groups

A classical trivalent bioisosteric replacement is –CH= with –N=

    a. This replacement when applied to cholesterol resulted in 20, 25-diazacholesterol which is a potent inhibitor of cholesterol biosynthesis. The greater electronegativity of the nitrogen atom could be responsible for the biological activity of this bioisostere.

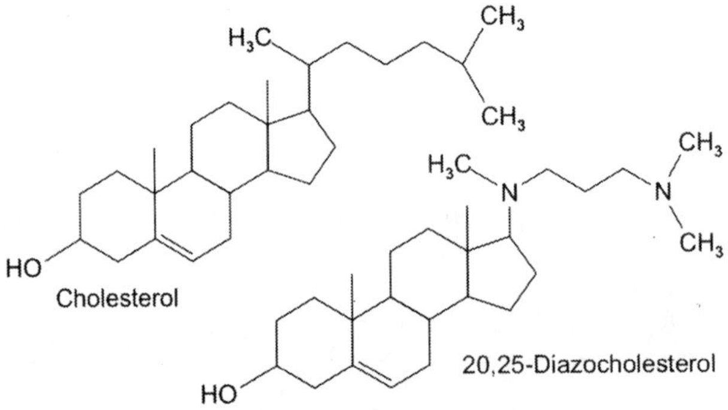

Cholesterol

20,25-Diazocholesterol

Cholesterol

    b. Aminopyrine was marketed as an analgesic and anti-inflammatory drug in 1896. In 1922, it was revealed that aminopyrine was a carcinogen. Propylphenazone,

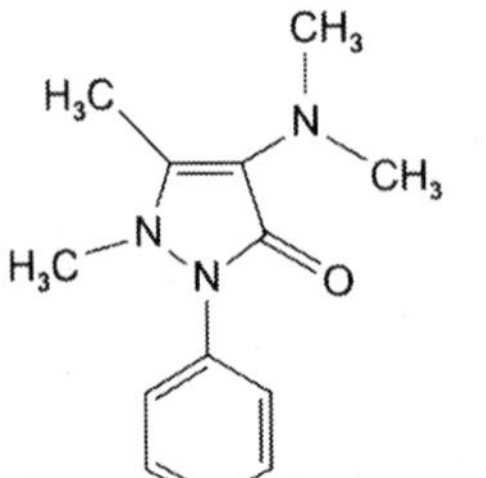

4-Dimethylamino antipyrine 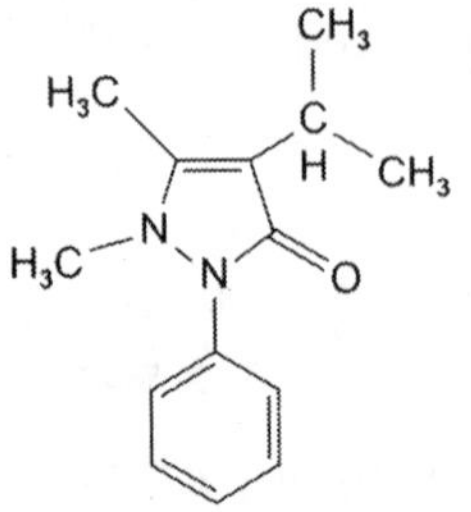   4-Isopropyl antipyrine

developed by Roche in 1951. The combination of propyphenazone, paracetamol and caffeine (trade name—Saridone) was indicated for the management of headache. The 4-dimethylamino-antipyrine and its carba-isostere are about equally active as antipyretics. At the same time, bioisosteric modification of dimethylamino group removed its carcinogenic action

Tetravalent Atoms and Groups

The cholinergic drug, acetylcholine was also developed into bio isosteric analogs in which tetravalent nitrogen was replaced by tetravalent phosphorous or arsenic but discarded due to more toxicity.

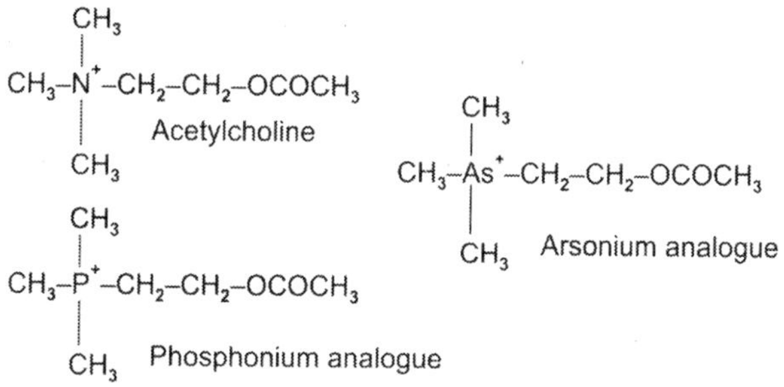

Acetylcholine

Arsonium analogue

Phosphonium analogue

Ring equivalents

a. In sulphonamide antibacterials, phenyl group may be replaced by heterocyclic group as in sulphadizine and sulmethoxazole. No difference in activity is observed between the original drug and its isostere.

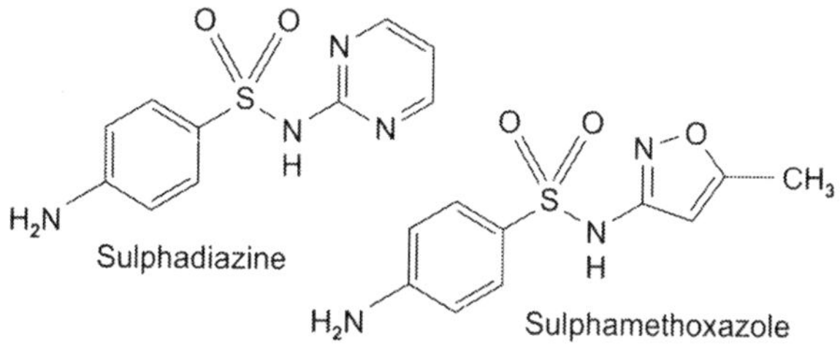

Sulphadiazine

Sulphamethoxazole

b. In arylthiazine-1, 1-dioxide, the replacement of benzene nucleus (e.g. piroxicam) with thienothiazine moiety gave tenoxicam. Both the drug act by the same mechanism, act on the same receptor are cyclooxygenase inhibitor. The only diiference is that in tenoxicam due to isosteric replacement, there is a long plasma half life.

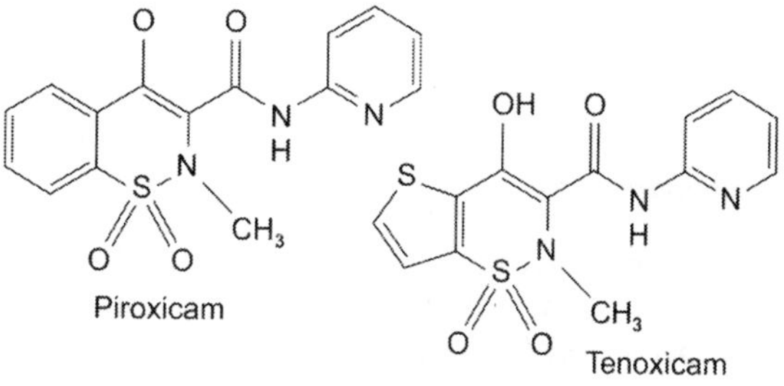

Piroxicam

Tenoxicam

Ramotodome produced nazatidinean antiulcerative drug, through bioisoteric modification.

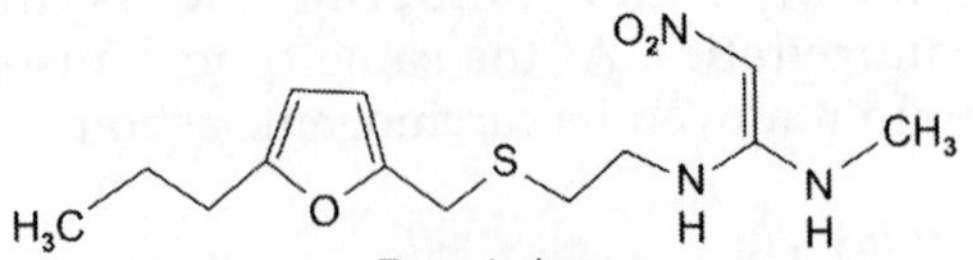

Ramotodome

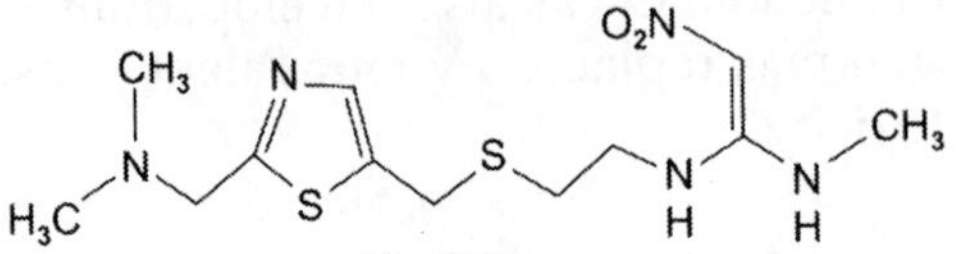

Nizatidine

The bioisosteric ring replacement in sildenafil produced verdenafil. It is more potent and more selective than sildenafil at inhibiting phosphodiesterase-5 enzyme.

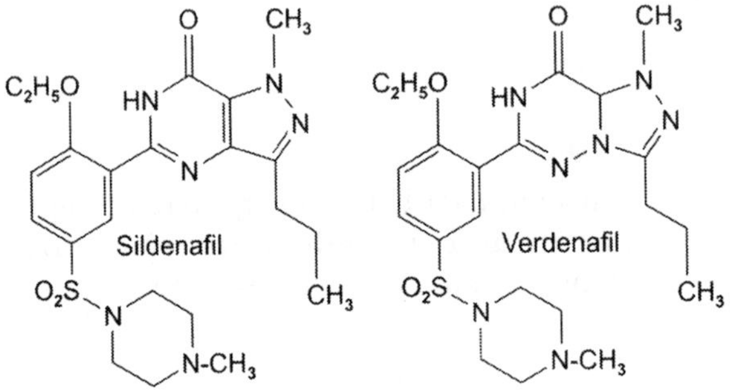

Sildenafil

Verdenafil

Bioisosters of Pyridine

The pyridine ring of nicotine can be replaced by other heterocyclic rings like methyl isoxazole or methyl isothiazole with similar activity.

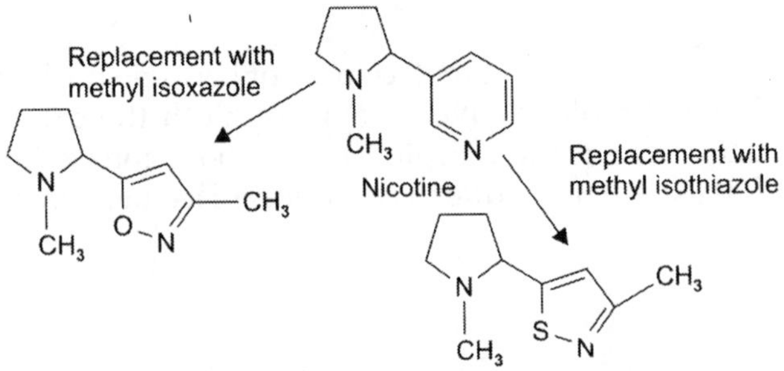

Replacement with methyl isoxazole

Nicotine

Replacement with methyl isothiazole

Bioisoteres of Other Heterocycles

Selective cyclooxygenase-2 inhibitors is a nice example of bioisoters of heterocycles. The comparison of celecoxib, etorocoxib and valdecoxib shows that isoxazoles, pyridines and pyrazoles are good bioisoters.

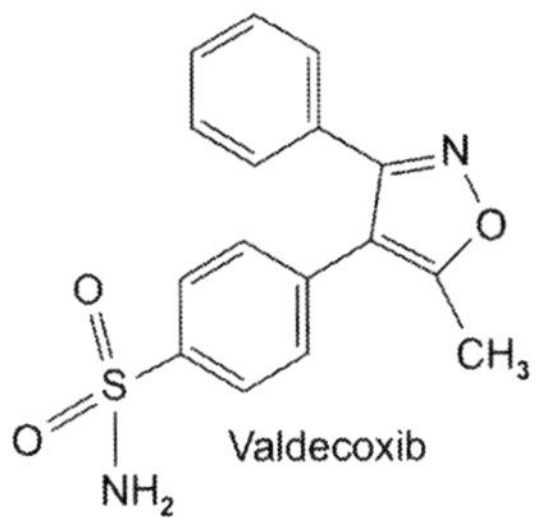

Valdecoxib

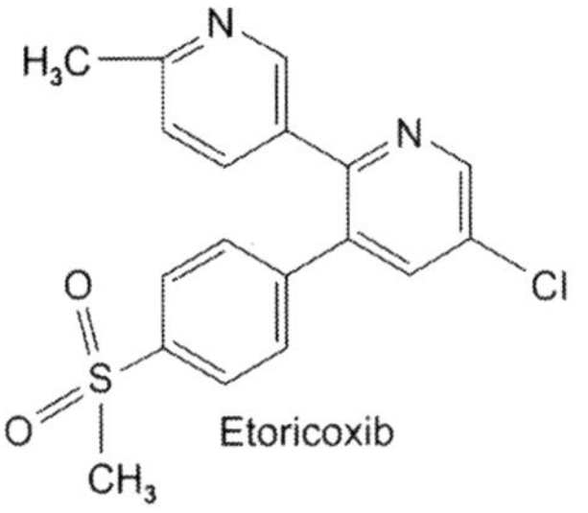

Etoricoxib

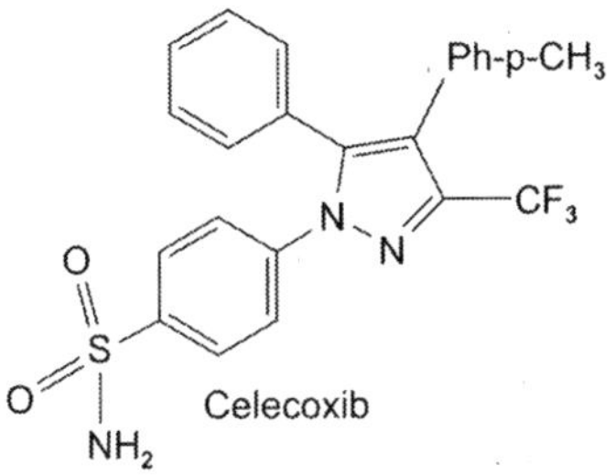

Celecoxib

NONCLASSIC BIOISOSTERISM

Cyclic and Noncyclic Bioisostere

Diethylstilbestrol is a noncyclic and nonsteroidal compound but it has similar activity as a female hormone, estradiol.

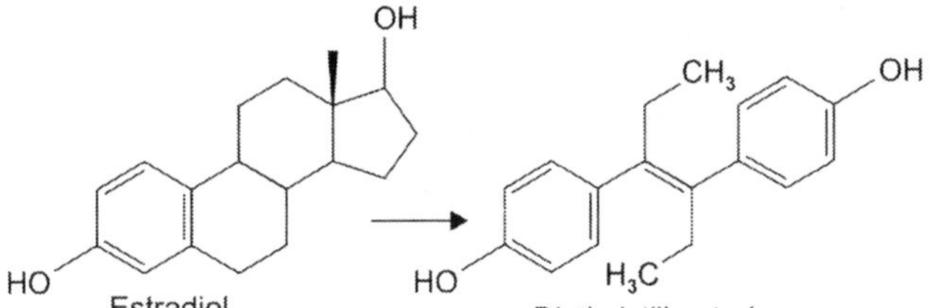

Estradiol

Diethylstilbestrol

Carboxylic Acid Bioisoters

There is a evidence of similarity between *p*-aminobenzoic acid and sulphanilamide . This similarity is based on electronic and conformational aspects as well as the physicochemical properties such as pKa and log *P*.

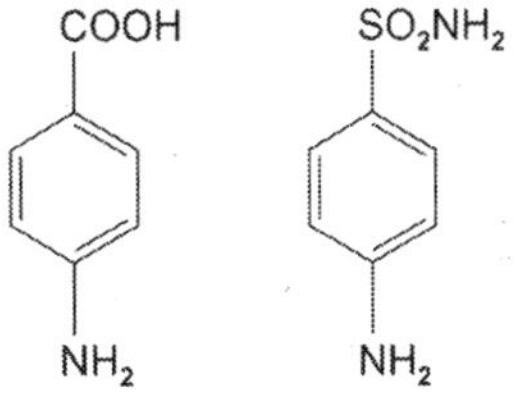

The replacement of –COOH in gamma amino butyric acid (GABA) by tetrazole group, resulting a tetrazole bioisostere of GABA, a potent antiepileptic agent.

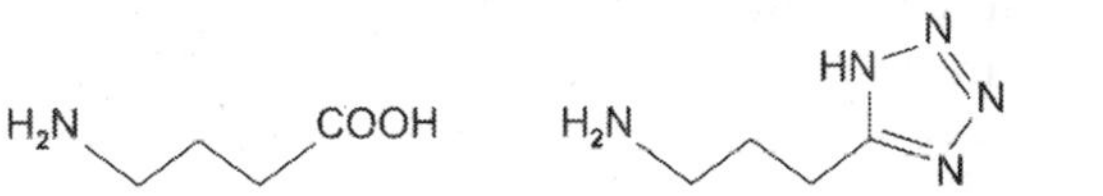

GABA

Tetrazole bioisostere of GABA

Hydroxyl Group Bioisosteres

Isoproterenol is a example of beta adrenoreceptor agonist, used as bronchodilator. In this 3-hydroxyl group has been replaced with bioisosteric groups which include albuterol (3-CH_2OH), soterenol (3-$NHSO_2CH_3$) and carbuterol (3-$NHCONH_2$). All of these compounds show potent and selective activities.

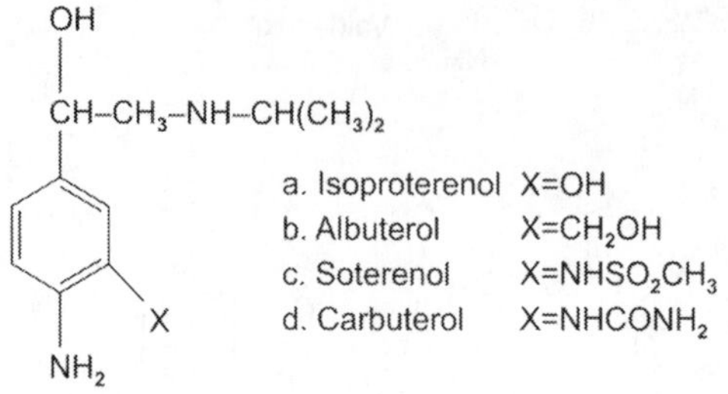

OH

CH–CH$_3$–NH–CH(CH$_3$)$_2$

a. Isoproterenol X=OH
b. Albuterol   X=CH$_2$OH
c. Soterenol   X=NHSO$_2$CH$_3$
d. Carbuterol   X=NHCONH$_2$

X

NH$_2$

Another example of the application of nonclassic bioisosterism can be illustrated by the discovery in 1957 of lidocaine from mepivacaine, contributing to the design of the important anesthetic agent with predominant anti arrhythmic properties.

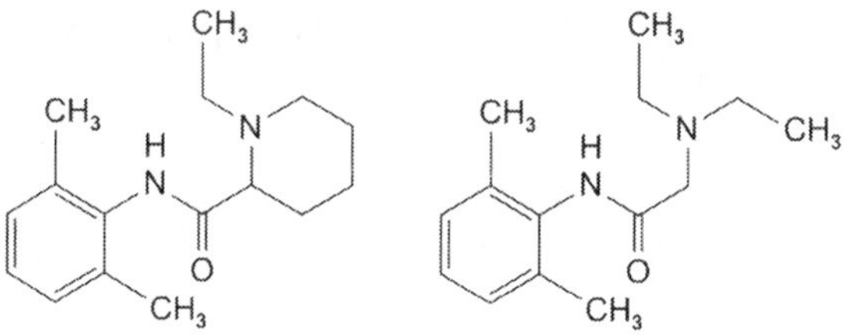

Mepivacaine

Lidocaine

Case Studies

Example 1
Interchange of hydroxyl and thiol groups

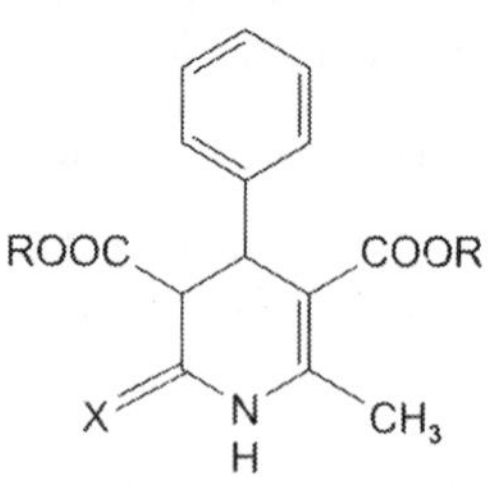

1,4-Dihydropyrimidine

In order to enhance the calcium channel blocking capacity of certain dihydropyrimidine agents, a number of isosteric analogues with the general structure were synthesized. Substitution of the hydroxyl with an amino resulted in analogues with similar potency. However, substitution with the thiol resulted in enhanced potency. This is due to the size of the substituent, described here as the van der Waal's radii and the hydrogen bonding ability. Therefore, replacement with the amino group, which has a similar size, resulted in similar potency and replacement with the sterically optimal thiol resulted in an analogue which was more potent (Table 3.4).

Compound	X	van der Waal's radius (Å)	$IC_{50}(nM)$
		Table 3.4: Calcium channel blocking activity of 1, 4-dihydropyrimidines	
1.	=O	1.40	140
2.	=NH	1.50	160
3.	=S	1.85	17

Example 2

Another classic example of isosteric replacement involving phenol (PhOH), can be found in the search for adrenergic derivatives, structurally related to catecholamines. This example illustrates the exchange of phenolic hydroxyl group present in compound 1 with the alkyl sulphonamide unit in compound 2, through the use of non-classic bioisosterism of functional groups. The results obtained on carrying out bioassays with these compounds, witness comparable biological activities through the mechanism of equivalent action, allowing us to conclude that both functional groups involved are authentic bioisosteres. This bioisosteric relationship was experimentally evidenced by determining the degree of acidity of these substances. Both compounds are of comparable acidity (pKA = 9.1 and 9.6 respectively), explaining the similarity of biological profile in function of equivalent interactions of both molecules with site receptor, possibly through ionic bonding, in the presence of a similar acidity or even through hydrogen bonding. Furthermore, both acidic groups, i.e. R-PhOH and $RPhNHSO_2CH_3$ are, in this case, monovalent groups. However, the identified bioisosteric relationship between the PhOH and $PhNHSO_2CH_3$ groups, confirmed for adrenergic derivatives 1 and 2, is not extensive to other bioreceptors in which the process of molecular recognition is distinct.

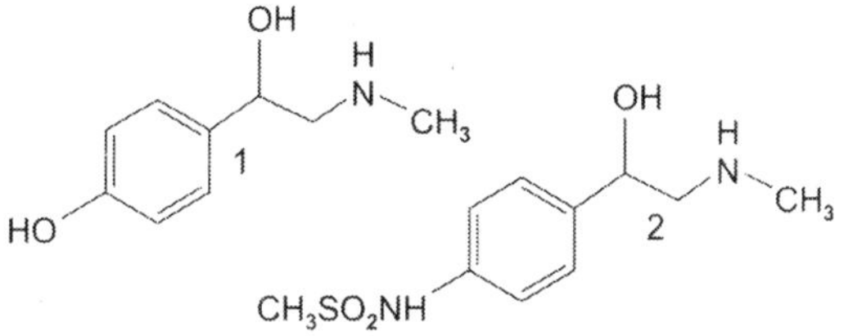

Example 3

The phenomenon of bioisosterism can be best demonstrated through an example of rofecoxib as a starting point. The bioisosteres for the lactone moiety was developed by specifying the replacement contain an aromatic carbon attached to the remaining phenyl group. The results (Fig. 3.1) contain an impressive range of bioisosteres from the 'obvious' – such as Valdecoxib and Parecoxib – to more interesting actives, such as an analogue of Etoricoxib. However, the results also contain 'nonobvious' bioisosteres such as the 12nM thiazolotriazole compound as shown in the Fig. 3.1.

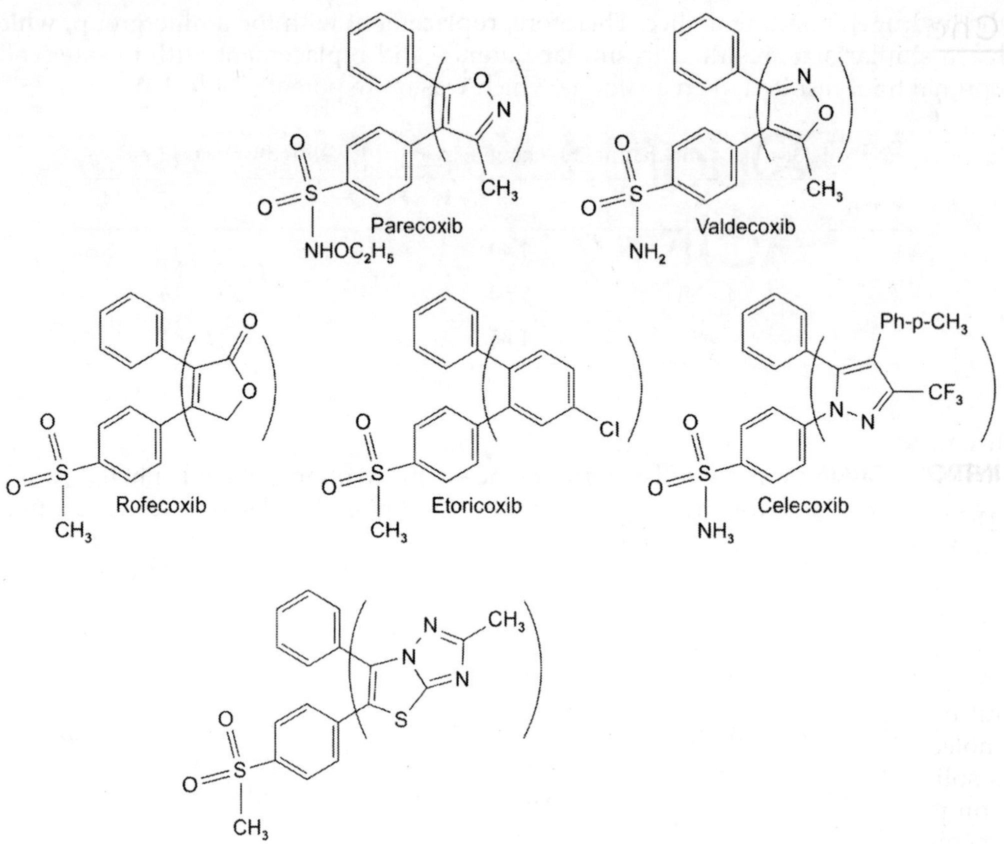

Fig. 3.1: Bioisosteric comparison of coxib derivatives

4

Quantitative Structure—Activity Relationship: Part I

INTRODUCTION

The behavior of a molecule can be predicted from its structure. For example, molecules containing one to four carbon atoms are gases at room temperature (methane CH_4, ethane C_2H_6, propane C_3H_8, butane C_4H_{10}). As more carbons are added, the substance becomes a liquid (hexane, a liquid, has six carbon atoms, C_6H_{14}) and finally a solid (octadecane, a solid, $C_{18}H_{38}$). If we add one oxygen atom to methane (CH_4), the molecule formed is a liquid we know as methanol (CH_3OH). As we add chlorine atoms, nitrogen atoms or any other atom, we can predict the effect of these additions on the molecule's behavior. This behavior is not limited to predicting whether the molecule is a solid, liquid or gas, but includes predicting how toxic or biologically active the compound will be. This field of science which combines the mathematics with chemistry is called *computational chemistry*. It deals with finding relationships called *quantitative structure–property relationship* (QSPR) or *quantitative structure activity–relationship* (QSAR).

QSAR, the commonly used terminology is based on structure–activity relation (SAR) approach. The QSAR is the study of how the physicochemical properties of a series of compounds affect their biological activity. The physiochemical properties or theoretical molecular descriptors for the chemicals or drug molecules are measured or calculated and these are related to biological activities using a mathematical equation.

Biological activity = F (physicochemical properties)

Biological activity is expressed as log $(1/C)$, where C is the minimum concentration required to cause a defined biological response. Other parameters for biological activity may be mathematical relationship in the form of equation between biological activity and measurable physicochemical parameters IC_{50}, ED_{50}, K_i, K_m, *etc.*

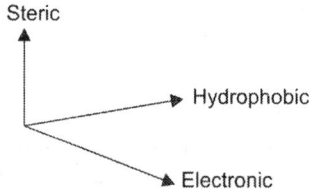

Physicochemical properties can be broadly classified into three general types:
* Electronic
* Steric
* Hydrophobic

In order to carry out traditional QSAR, a range of analogues is synthesized which have common skeleton, but which have different substituents. The activities of these analogues are measured and a formula is worked out relating these biological activities to the physical properties considered to be important (e.g. size, hydrophobicity, electronegativity, dipole moment, hydrogen bonding ability, *etc.*). Several of these properties are likely to influence activity and it would be ideal if one could synthesize analogues where one physical property was varied independently of any other. However, this is rarely possible. Changing one substituent for another usually results in several physical properties being altered at the same time. This also makes it difficult to identify whether one physical property is more important to activity than another. Therefore, in order to make sense of the data, it is necessary to make use of suitable computer software programme. Intuition alone is not enough.

There are several reasons why the physical properties of a compound should be important to biological activity. The overall hydrophobic character of a compound influences how efficiently it can cross cell membranes; the hydrophobic character and size of individual substituents may influence how well the compound interact and fits into its binding site, while the electronic character of substituents can influence the basicity of the compound, affecting both absorption and receptor binding. These are just a few of the factors that have to be taken into consideration.

Procedure

There are many software programs that help in deriving equations, but it is up to the medicinal chemist to decide what data to put in. Clearly, the biological activity of each compound has to be included, but the chemist has to decide which physical features might be more important to biological activity. Then derive an equation to test whether they really are important. QSAR is not a case of putting as much data as one can into a computer and hoping that the machine will make sense of it all. In fact, it is usually best to derive an initial equation based on only one or two physical feature. Hopefully, the initial equation will give calculated activities close to the experimentally measured activities, but there will almost certainly be compounds which don't obey the mathematical equation-outriders. Such compounds should not be viewed as 'nuisance' quite the opposite in fact. The medicinal chemist can study these molecules and try to identify a physical feature which these molecules have which the others don't, then search for a more advanced formula that includes that property. QSAR equations constantly evolve and it is the medicinal chemist who directs that evolution.

Certain physical properties are almost always considered in a QSAR equation. These are the hydrophobicity (or fatty character) of the molecule and/or its substituents, the electronic properties of its substituents and size of its substituents.

Hydrophobicity Parameter

There are two parameters, which are commonly used to relate drug absorption and distribution with biological activity: (1) Hydrophobicity (2) Hydrophobicity substituent constant (π). The former parameter refers to the whole molecule while the latter is related to substituent groups. A drug molecule has to pass through a number of biological membranes to reach at the site of action.

Hydrophobicity is the parameter to use as a measure of the movement of drug through these membranes. Hydrophobicity is a partitioning of the compound between an aqueous and non-aqueous phase. The hydrophobicity of a molecule is normally measured by its **log P** value, where P is known as the partition coefficient. P can be measured experimentally by measuring the relative solubility of a compound in an aqueous and non-aqueous phase (e.g. octanol-water system) where

$$P = \frac{\text{Conc. of compound in octanol}}{\text{Conc. of compound in water}}$$

The more hydrophobic the compound is, the greater proportion of it will dissolve in the organic layer, and the higher the value of P or log P.

With most drugs, *in vivo* activity increase as the log P value increases. In other words, activity increases with increasing hydrophobicity. This is usually an indication that increasing hydrophobicity allows easier passage of the drug through cell membranes in order to reach target site. This might imply that one could keep increasing activity by continually increasing hydrophobicity. In fact, this is not the case. Most of the QSAR experiments are carried out on compounds that have a limited range of log P values (e.g. Eqs (4.1)–(4.4). In this case, straight line is obtained.

$$\log 1/C = K_1 \log P + K_2 \tag{4.1}$$

where K_1 and K_2 are constant.

If compounds were synthesized with a much broader range of log P values, an optimum log P value would be found beyond which activity would fall. A parabolic curve (Fig. 4.1) would be the result having the formula:

$$\log (\text{activity}) = -k_1 (\log P)^2 + k_2 \log P + k_3 \tag{4.2}$$

where k_1, k_2 and k_3 are constants.

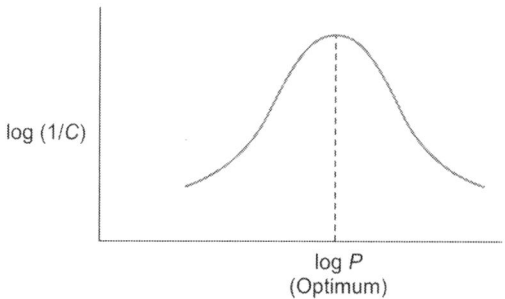

Fig. 4.1: Parabolic curve relating log (activity) vs log P

Looking at Eq. (4.2), the $-(\log P)^2$ entry has a negative effect on activity, whereas the log P entry has positive effect. When P is low, log P is more important than $-(\log P)^2$. Therefore, in the first part of the curve, log P is more significant and activity increases as log P increases. In second part of the curve, the $-(\log P)^2$ factor becomes dominant and activity falls.

Log P is present in most of the QSAR equations involving *in vivo* activity, since activity is dependent on drugs crossing membranes. If activity is measured by in vitro tests, the log P factor may be less significant and may even be absent.

Substituent Hydrophobicity Constant or p-substituent Constant

The partition coefficients describe the overall hydrophobicity of a molecule, but it is also possible to quantify the hydrophobic character of individual substituents using sets of tables that give hydrophobicity constant (π) for each substituent. The substituent hydrophobicity constant is a measure of how hydrophobic substituent is, relative to hydrogen. The value is measured experimentally by comparing the log P values of a compound with and without the substituents. The hydrophobicity constant (π) for the substituent's (X) is then obtained using the following equation:

$$\pi_X = \log P_X - \log P_H \tag{4.3}$$

where P_H is the partition coefficient for standard compound, and P_X is the partition coefficient for analogue containing the substituent 'X'. If π is positive then the substituents is more hydrophobic than hydrogen and drug will favor the non aqueous phase. If π is negative, then the substituent is less hydrophobic than hydrogen and drug will favor the aqueous phase.

It may not seen obvious why this would be useful if one has already measured the hydrophobicity of the molecule as a whole. However, there are two reasons why such constants can be useful. First of all, hydrophobicity constants can be used to calculate log P values for different compounds, avoiding the need to measure each log P value experimentally. For example, the log P value for *para*-bromoanisole can be calculated as 2.97, given the log P value for benzene (2.13) and π constants for bromine and methoxy (0.86 and –0.02 respectively).

log P = 2.13   Log P = 2.13 + 0.86 – 0.02
= 0.97

The π constants are only truly relevant for the structures that were used to determine them. Therefore, the aromatic π constants are relevant for substituted benzene, but are less reliable for heteroatomic ring systems. Similarly, the aromatic π constants are not relevant for aliphatic substituents and there is a separate table of constants for the latter. Ideally, accurate π values should be obtained for the molecular skeleton being studied. However, this may not always be possible and the values derived from different systems may need to be used as an approximation.

The second reason π values can be useful in QSAR is that they might be introduced into QSAR equation itself to identify whether hydrophobic substituents at particular parts of the molecular skeleton have any localized influence on activity. In fact, it is perfectly possible for a QSAR equation to calculate both log P and π. The former measures how the hydrophobic character of the molecule as a whole influences activity through such factors as the ability to cross cell membranes, while the latter demonstrates any localized hydrophobic influences that are at work. For example, the discovery that hydrophobic substituents at the *para* position of an aromatic ring are beneficial to activity might indicate that there is a hydrophobic binding pocket in the binding site that can accommodate such substituents.

Electronic Parameters

The electronic properties of different substituent present in a drug molecule can also play an important role in affecting biological activity. In a generalized way, non-polar and polar drugs in the unionized form are readily transported through membranes than polar drug and drugs in their ionized form. Furthermore, once the drug reaches at the target site, the distribution of electron in its structure will control the type of bonds it form with that target which in turn affects its biological activity. In other words, the electron distribution in a drug molecule will have an effect on how strongly that drug binds to its target site, which in turn affects its activity. The distribution of electron within a molecule depends on the nature of electron withdrawing and electron donating groups found in that structure. The electronic properties of aromatic substituent are described by the **Hammett substitution constant, σ.**

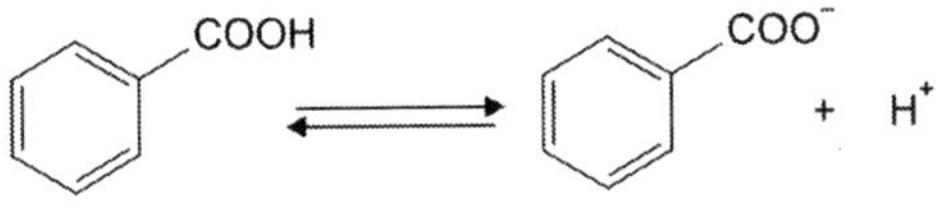

Benzoic acid

These constants are shown in Table 4.1 and were measured experimentally by measuring what effect the substituents had on the dissociation of benzoic acids. Benzoic acid itself is a weak acid and only partially ionizes in water. Equilibrium is set up between the ionized and nonionized forms, where the relative proportion of these

Table 4.1 *Physiochemical parameters used in QSAR investigations*

Substituent	π	σ_m	σ_p	E_s
-H	0.00	0.00	0.00	0.0
-CH$_3$	0.56	−0.07	−0.17	−1.2
-CH$_2$CH$_3$	1.02	−0.07	−0.15	−1.3
-CH$_2$CH$_2$CH$_3$	1.55	−0.07	−0.13	−1.6
-CH(CH$_3$)$_2$	1.53	−0.07	−0.15	−1.7
-OCH$_3$	−0.02	0.12	−0.27	−0.5
-Phenyl	1.96	0.06	−0.01	−3.8
-NH$_2$	−1.23	−0.16	−0.66	−0.6
-F	0.14	0.34	0.06	−0.4
-Cl	0.71	0.37	0.23	−0.9
-Br	0.86	0.39	0.23	−1.1
-I	1.12	0.35	0.18	−1.4
-CF$_3$	0.88	0.43	0.54	−2.4
-OH	−0.67	0.12	−0.37	−0.5
-COCH$_3$	−0.55	0.38	0.50	−1.5[1]
-COOCH$_3$[1]	0.01	0.50	0.56	−1.8
-NHCOCH$_3$	−0.97	0.21	0.00	−2.8[1]
-NO$_2$	−0.28	0.71	0.78	−2.5
-CN	−0.57	0.56	0.66	−0.5
-N+(CH$_3$)$_3$	−0.25	0.78	0.50	−2.3[1]
-COOH	−0.16	0.36	0.45	−1.4[1]

species is known as equilibrium or **dissociation constants** K_H (the subscript H signifies that there are no substituents on the aromatic ring):

$$K_H = \frac{[PhCOO^-]}{[PhCOOH]}$$

Substituents on the aromatic ring affect this equilibrium. Electron withdrawing group will stabilize the carboxylate anion and the equilibrium will shift to the ionized form and result in a larger equilibrium constant. An electron donating group will destabilize the carboxylate ion such that the equilibrium shifts to the left and results in a smaller equilibrium constant. The Hammett substituent constant (σ_x) for a particular substituent (X) is defined by the following equation:

$$\sigma_X = \log \frac{K_X}{K_H} = \log K_X - \log K_H \qquad (4.4)$$

As with hydrophobic constants, these constants are only accurate for the molecular structures from which they are derived. Electron withdrawing substituents (e.g. Cl, CN, CF_3 have positive σ values due to induction effect. When the phenol group is at the *para* position, σ_p is −0.37 reflecting the fact that the group is now electron donating at that position due to CF_3) have positive σ values while electron donating substituent (e.g. CH_3, CH_2CH_3) have negative σ values (Fig. 4.2). The value of the Hammett substituent takes into account both the substituent's inductive and resonance effects, and so the value depends on whether the substituents is *meta* or *para* to rest of the molecule (σ_m and σ_p). For example, σ_m for a phenol group is 0.12, reflecting the electron withdrawing influence felt at the *meta* position due to resonance effect. It should be noted that aromatic substitution constants for *ortho* substitution are unreliable since *ortho* substituent can have a steric as well as an electronic effect.

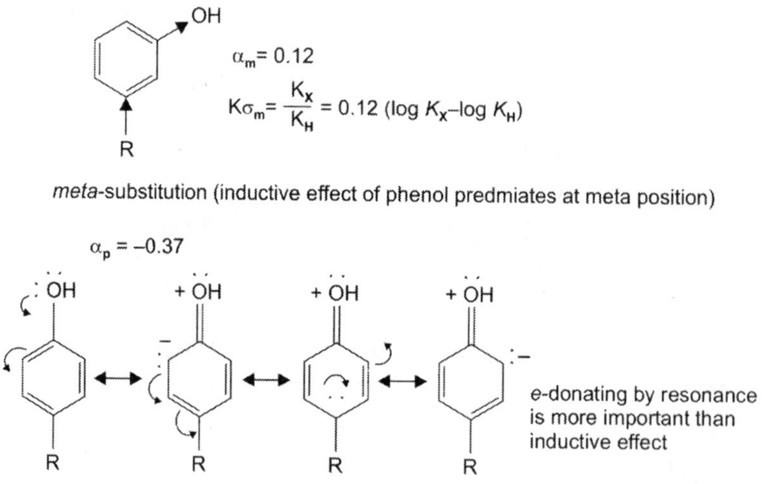

$$\alpha_m = 0.12$$
$$K\sigma_m = \frac{K_X}{K_H} = 0.12 \ (\log K_X - \log K_H) \qquad (4.5)$$

meta-substitution (inductive effect of phenol predmiates at meta position)

$$\alpha_p = -0.37$$

e-donating by resonance is more important than inductive effect

Fig. 4.2: Electronic influence of a phenol at meta and para position

Other constants which separately quantify are the inductive effect (F) or the resonance effect (R) of aromatic substituent.

Aliphatic electronic substituents constants have been obtained by measuring the rate of hydrolysis for a series of aliphatic esters, where methyl ethanoate is the parent ester.

The extent to which the rate of hydrolysis is affected is a measure of the substituent's electronic effect, which arises purely from inductive effects. Electron donating groups reduce the rate of hydrolysis and therefore have negative values. Electron withdrawing groups increase the rate of hydrolysis and have positive values. Bulky substituents may also have a steric effect on the rate of hydrolysis by shielding the ester from attack. It is possible to separate out these two effects by measuring hydrolysis rates under basic and acidic conditions. Under basic conditions, steric and electronic factors are important, whereas under acidic condition only steric factors are important. By comparing the rates, values for the electronic effect (σ), and for the steric effect (E_s) (see below) can be determined.

$$\text{Hydrolysis}$$
$$X-CH_2-CO-OCH_3 \longrightarrow X-CH_2-CO-OH + CH_3OH$$
$$\text{Aliphatic ester} \qquad\qquad \text{Aliphatic acid}$$

Steric Factor

In order for a drug to bind effectively to the target site, the dimension of the pharmacophore of the drug must be complementary to those of target site. It is a measure of the bulkiness of the group it represents and it effects on the closeness of contact between the drug and receptor site. It is hard to quantitate. The size of different substituents can clearly be important to the activity of compounds. Bulky groups may lower activity by preventing drugs from fitting properly into the binding sites. On the other hand, bulky substituent may increase activity by forcing a compound to adopt the required active conformation for binding. Measuring the steric properties of substituents is not as straightforward as the measurement of a substituent's hydrophobic or electronic character. However, there are three methods that are generally used:

i. **Taft's steric factor** is a measure of a substituent's size and is determined experimentally by measuring the effect on the rate of a chemical reaction. Different substituents have varied effect on the rate of a chemical reaction carried out on the parent structure. Large substituents next to reaction center hinder the reaction more than smaller substituents, so difference in reaction rate lead to a measure of a substituent's size.

ii. **Molar refractivity (MR)** is a measure of the volume occupied by an atom or group-equation includes the molecular weight (MW), density (d), and the index of refraction(n). It is calculated as per below given formula:

$$MR = \frac{(n^2-1)}{(n^2+2)} \times \frac{MW}{d}$$

The term MW/d defines a volume while the $(n^2-1)/(n^2+2)$ term provides correction factor by defining how easily the substituents can be polarized. This is particularly significant if the substituent has π electrons or lone pairs of electrons.

iii. A third method of determining size is to use a computer software program called **Sterimol** which calculates steric factors known as **Verloop steric parameters**. This program measures the standard bond angles, Vander Walls radii, bond length, and possible conformations for the substituents. The advantage of this approach is that Verloop steric parameter can be calculated for any substituents without the need for any experimental measurements. For example, the Verloop steric parameters for a carboxylic acid group are shown in Fig. 4.3. L is the length of the substituents while B_1–B_4 is the radii of the group.

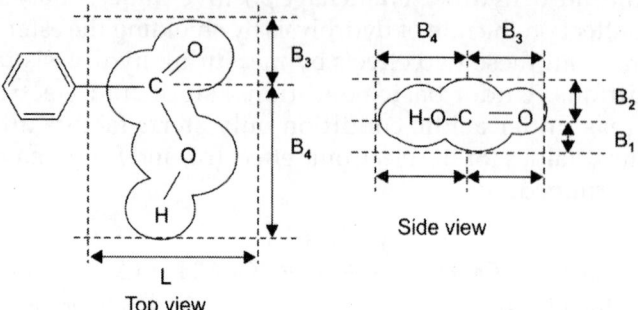

Fig. 4.3: Verloop steric parameters for a carboxylic acid

Hansch Equation

It is proposed that drug action could be divided into 2 stages: (1) Transport and (2) Binding each of these stages depend upon the physical and chemical properties of the drug.

The Hansch equation is the QSAR equation that relates physicochemical properties to biological activity. Typically, these equations will include a variety of parameters, the most common being log P, π, σ, MR, and E_s. For example, a typical Hansch equation would have the following format.

$$\log \frac{1}{C} = - k_1 (\log P)^2 + k_2 \log P + k_3 \pi + k_4 \sigma + k_5 E_s + k_6 \tag{4.6}$$

where k_1–k_6 are constants. These constants would be determined by computer in order to get the best fitting line. Activity is often measured by $1/C$, where C is the concentration of a drug required to produce a specific effect (e.g. the concentration required to produce 50% inhibition of an enzyme). The more active the drug, the smaller the concentration required, and the larger the value of $1/C$.

An example of a Hansch equation is shown here with the inhibitory activity of a series of substituted *N*-(Phenoxyethyl) cyclopropylamines against the enzyme, **monoamine oxidase**. This shows that hydrophobic substituents that are electron withdrawing are good for activity.

$$\log \frac{1}{C} = 0.398 \, \pi + 1.089 \, \sigma + 1.03 \, E_s + 4.541 \tag{4.7}$$

The $E_{s\,(3,5)}$, factor represents the Taft steric parameters of any substituents which are at the meta position. This shows that bulky groups are bad for activity since such groups have a negative Es value.

It should be appreciated that a QSAR equation is only as good as the data that has been entered. Usually, a range of compounds are synthesized to quantify the effect that two or three physical parameters (e.g. π and σ) have on biological activity. However, it is crucial to choose a valid set of compounds in order to carry out the analysis. This means that the substituents present must give a good range of values for the physical parameters concerned, but they must also distinguish between the parameters such that they are not correlated (i.e. follow the same trend). For example, consider the substituent F, Cl, Br and I, where I is most electron withdrawing and F is least electron withdrawing. However, the hydrophobic character of these substituents also increases in the same sequence. Therefore, there is no way of knowing whether any similar trend in biological activity is due to the hydrophobic or the electronic properties of the substituents. In order to identify suitable substituents for QSAR studies, it is useful to consult **Craig plots**.

Craig Plots

Craig plots compare two separate physical properties for different substituents. The example in Fig. 4.4 compares the σ and π properties of different substituents by plotting the σ values on the y axis and the π-values on the x-axis.

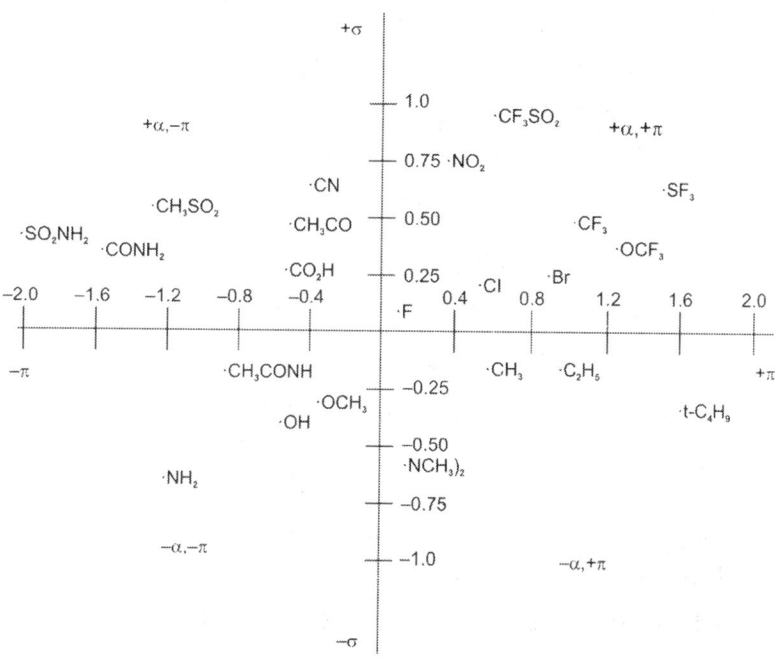

Fig. 4.4: Craig plot comparing σ and π

The plot reveals group that are similar with respect to both the properties and those that are not included. For example, a cyano group and a methyl ketone group have similar π and σ values, whereas a cyano and trifluoromethyl group has similar σ values but quite different π values.

Plots such as these are extremely important in deciding which substituent should be used in a QSAR study when one wants to distinguish between two physical properties such as σ and π. Ideally, the compounds studied should contain substituents from all four quadrants of the plot. Therefore, choosing analogues with the substituents Cl, Br, CF_3 and NO_2 (all from the same quadrant) would not allow the derivation of a valid QSAR equation since it would be difficult to tell whether variation in activity are due to σ or π. Substituents such as Cl, CF_3, Ethyl, OH and CN would be more valid.

Other Factors

Other physicochemical factors can be introduced into the Hansch equation to try and improve the correlation between structure and biological activity. For example, QSAR equations have been derived which measure how the orientation of a dipole moment affects biological activity. Other QSAR equations have been derived which relate molecular orbital to activity.

Free Wilson Analysis

Free Wilson proposed a model, which is also called *de novo* model, which says that the biological activity of a compound is the sum of the contributions of all the substituents and the parent moiety.

It is true structure–activity relationship model. It is based on the following assumption:

- The entire drug listed should have the same parent structure.
- The substitution pattern in various derivatives has to be same.
- The substitutions have to contribute to the biological activity additively and in the same position with a constant amount being independent of the presence or absence of other substitution in the molecules (Fig. 4.5).

So the total activity (*A*) of a certain derivative is the sum of constant independent partial contribution.

$$A = \Sigma\,(ai\,I\,i) + \mu \tag{4.8}$$

where, I = the substituent, ai = the contribution of substituent I, Ii = the contribution of parent structure and 'μ' is the average activity. The equation is solved by multilinear regression using the presence (1) or absence (0) of the different substituents as independent dummy parameters, while the measured activity served as the dependant variable. There is no need for any physicochemical parameters.

Fujita and Ban suggested two modifications in Free Wilson model. Biological activity was converted to log (1/C) or an equivalent terms like in Hansch analysis. Also μ is the activity of unsubstituted parent molecule instead of average activity. Today, Fujita-Ban modified model has almost replaced the original Free Wilson model. Kubinyi has combined Hansch and Free-Wilson model as mixed approach. But a general criticism of Free Wilson method is that it is too simplified and does not offer any advantage to medicinal chemist. The assumption that the substituents are independent is not always correct. Another limitation is that the information obtained cannot be used for other substituents which were not present in the original set. The main advantage of Free

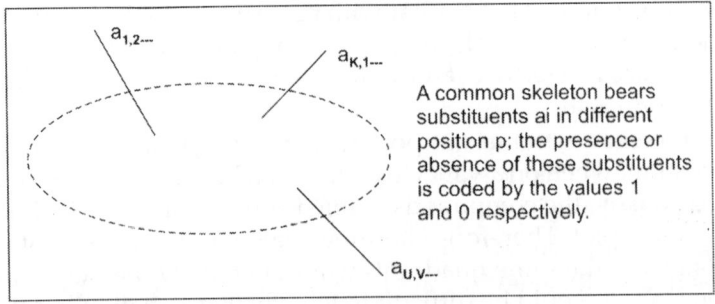

Fig. 4.5: Schematic presentation of molecule for Free Wilson analysis

Wilson method is that it can be incorporated into Hansch analysis by using an indicator variable (I). Many times, the chemist by intuition recognizes the importance of a substituent. In such cases an indicator variable (I) can be used in Hansch equation, where $I = 1$ if a substituent is present, and $I =$ zero if absent.

Equation (4.9) describes the antiadrenergic activities for 22 different *m-*, *p-* and *ṁ, p-* disubstituted analogs of the N, N dimethyl-α-bromophenylamine (Fig. 4.6), where C is the concentration that causes a 50% reduction of the adrenergic effect of a certain epinephrine dose.

$$\log 1/C = -0.301\ (\pm0.50)\ [m\text{-F}] + 0.27\ (\pm0.29)\ [m\text{-Cl}] + 0.434\ (\pm0.27)\ [m\text{-Br}] +$$
$$0.579\ (\pm0.50)\ [m\text{-I}] + 0.454\ (\pm0.27)\ [m\text{-Me}] + 0.340\ (\pm0.30)\ [p\text{-F}] + 0.768$$
$$(\pm0.30)\ [p\text{-Cl}] + 1.020\ (\pm0.30)\ [p\text{-Br}] + 1.429\ (\pm0.50)\ [p\text{-I}] + 1.256\ (\pm0.33)$$
$$[p\text{-Me}] + 7.821\ (\pm0.27) \tag{4.9}$$

(where $n = 22$; $r^2 = 0.94$; $s = 0.194$; $F = 16.99$)

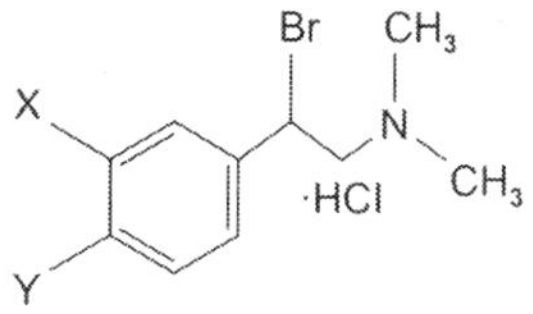

Fig. 4.6: *N, N*-dimehyl-α-bromo phenylamines

where n = number of compounds; r = correlation coefficient, measure for the relative quality of a model; s = standard deviation, measure for the absolute quality of a model; F = Fisher value, measure for statistical significance; C = molar concentration that causes a certain biological effect.

Equation (4.9) illustrates the main advantage of Free Wilson analysis: only the biological activity values and the chemical structure of the compounds need to be known to derive a QSAR model. On the other hand Free Wilson analysis has several shortcomings:

a. At least two different position of substituents must be chemically modified;
b. Predictions can only be made for new combination of substituents already included in the analysis;
c. Single point determination, i.e. the single occurrence of a certain structural feature in the whole data set obscure the statistical results;
d. Many degrees of freedom are wasted to describe every substituent.

Nevertheless, Free Wilson analysis is often used to see at a glance which physicochemical properties might be important for the biological activity. In this data set, it can be easily concluded from Eq. (4.9) that:

• Biological activities increase with increasing lipophilicity (F to Cl, Br and I);
• Biological activities increase with electron donor properties (methyl has larger group contributions than the equilipophilic, Cl);
• *meta*-substituents have lower group contributions than *para*-substituents.

Note: A negative coefficient indicates that the presence of that group is unfavorable to activity; a positive coefficient indicates that the presence of that group is favourable to activity.

Topliss Schemes

This approach is completely non mathematical and non statistical and does not need computerization of the data. The Topliss scheme is useful in planning which analogues to synthesize if compounds are being synthesized and tested one at time. There is Topliss scheme for aromatic substituent (Fig. 4.7). The scheme is designed to rationalize differences in activity based factors that we already discussed: the hydrophobic, electronic and steric factors.

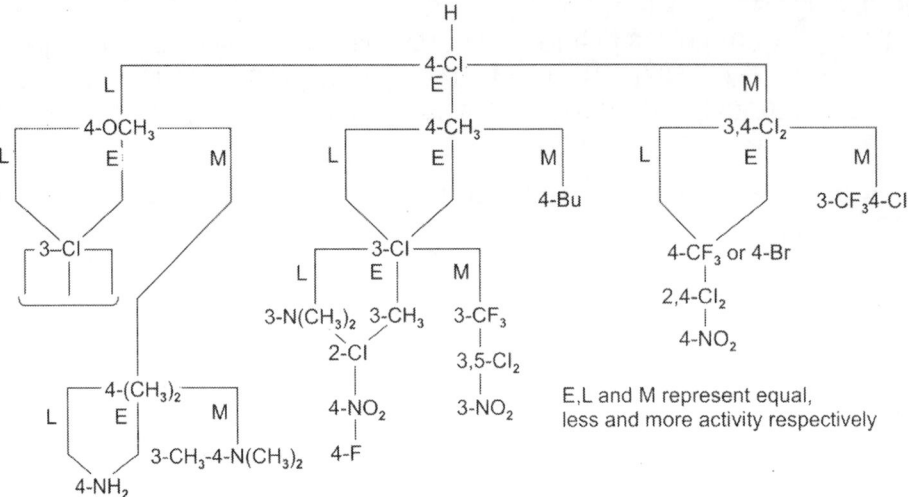

Fig. 4.7: Topliss scheme for aromatic substitutions

In order to use the Topliss scheme for aromatic substituents, the lead compound has to have an aromatic ring. The first analogue to be synthesized would then be 4-chloro analogue. The Chloro group is hydrophobic and electron withdrawing. If the activity of the chloro analogue proves to be greater than the lead compound, it is assumed that both of these properties are important, and so a second chloro group is introduced at the *meta* position to enhance both effects.

If the activity of the 4-chloro analogue drops, it suggests that both properties are bad for activity and so a more polar electron donating group (OCH_3) is placed at that instead. If activity drops again, it suggest that para substitution may be bad for steric reasons, and so a *meta*-chloro group is tried. On the other hand, if activity improves, further substituents are tried to determine the relative importance of hydrophobic and electronic properties.

The third possibility is that the activity of the 4-chloro derivative is similar to the lead compound in which case hydrophobicity may be good for activity, but an electron donating hydrophobic group (CH_3) would then be tried to test this theory out. Progress through the 'tree' is then continued based on similar arguments regarding the hydrophobic, electronic and steric properties of the substituents involved.

Quantitative Structure–Activity Relationship: Part II

INTRODUCTION

Quantitative structure–activity relationship (QSAR), in simplest terms, is a method for building computational or mathematical models to find out a possible statistically significant correlation between structure and function using a chemometric technique.

COMPARISON OF QSAR WITH SAR

1. QSAR is a mathematical relationship between the biological activities and measurable physiochemical parameter. In contrast, structure–activity relationship (SAR) is a relationship between the chemical or 3D structure of a molecule and its biological activities.
2. QSAR is mainly helpful in drug design. SAR is a valuable information in drug discovery and development. It is used for discovering and developing new compounds, as well as assessing potential health risks posed by existing compounds. For instance, the analysis of SAR enables the determination of which chemical groups play an important role in promoting a target effect in the organism. This determination allows rationally modification of the effect or improving the potency of a bioactive compound by changing its chemical structure or insert new chemical groups. In the case of risk assessment, similar data from the most sensitive toxicological endpoints can be used such as carcinogenicity or cardiotoxicity.
3. QSAR optimizes the properties of a lead compound. SAR is mainly done by lead molecule.
4. Quantitative SAR (QSAR) model is regarded as a special case of SAR (when relationships become quantified), and this model relates a set of *predictor* variables (x) to the potency of the response variable (Y) to predict the activity of chemicals. The unique methods allow researchers to go beyond merely characterizing structures as *active* or *inactive*, but predict the level of biological activity or potency. Overall, QSAR is a special case of SAR while SAR is not the special case of QSAR.

OBJECTIVES OF QSAR

Mostly, all the QSAR methods focus on the following goals:
- To quantitatively correlate and recapitulate the relationships between trends in chemical structure alterations and respective changes in biological activity (endpoint) for comprehending which chemical properties are most likely determinants for their biological activities

- To optimize the existing leads so as to improve their biological activities
- To predict the biological activities of untested and sometimes yet unavailable compounds

RATIONALE BEHIND QSAR MODELING

The extent of reliability in opting for QSAR modeling depends on the type or nature of property being predicted, the stage of the project and the relative ease and cost of compound synthesis and subsequent testing. More often QSAR models provide useful predictions but many times they fail, despite of good statistics generated from internal data used in training. Regardless of all such problems, QSAR becomes a useful alternative because of the following reasons:

- Conventional synthesis methods are expensive and time-consuming
- Biological assays are also too costly, often requires longer time, sacrifice of animals, or compounds in their pure forms
- Drug failures due to poor ADMET profiles at later stages of development (or even after commercialization) are exceedingly expensive and painful
- Large number of compounds are available due to combinatorial chemistry and high–throughput screening (HTS) approaches, but estimations are required for prioritization of synthesis and screening

EVOLUTION OF QSAR

QSAR methods originated way back in the nineteenth century. The chronological order in which these methods (1D and 2D QSAR) have evolved over a period of time is being given in Table 5.1.

Table 5.1: A brief history of earlier QSAR methodologies	
Researcher (Year)	*Contributions/Postulates*
Crum-Brown and Fraser (1868)	Physiological activities of substances could be correlated with their chemical composition and constitution, but they did not show how to represent the chemical structure in a quantitative manner
Richardson (1868)	Expressed the chemical structure as a function of solubility
Mills (1884)	Developed a Quantitative Structure Property Relationship (QSPR) model for the prediction of melting and boiling points in homologous series, results were accurate to better than one degree
Richet (1893)	Correlated toxicities of a set of alcohols, ethers and ketones with aqueous solubility and showed that their cytotoxicities are inversely related to their corresponding water solubilities
Overton and Meyer (1897, 1899)	Correlated partition coefficients of a group of organic compounds with their anesthetic potencies and concluded that narcotic (depressant) activity is dependent on the lipophilicity of the molecules
Hammett (1935, 1937)	Correlated the effect of the addition of a substituent on benzoic acid with the dissociation constant, postulated electronic sigma-rho constants and established the linear free-energy relationship (LFER) principle

(Contd.)

Table 5.1: A brief history of earlier QSAR methodologies

Researcher (Year)	*Contributions/Postulates*
Ferguson (1939)	Correlated depressant action with the relative saturation of volatile compounds in their vehicle and introduced a thermodynamic generalization to the toxicity
Bell and Roblin (1942)	Studied antibacterial activities of a series of sulphanilamides in terms of their ionizations
Albert (1948)	Examined the effects of ionization/electron distribution and steric access on the potencies of a multitude of aminoacridines
Taft (1952)	Postulated a method for separating polar, steric, and resonance effects and introduced the first steric parameter, E_S
Hansch and Muir (1962)	Correlated the biological activities of plant growth regulators with Hammett constants and hydrophobicity
Hansch and Fujita (1964)	Combined the hydrophobic constants with Hammett's electronic constants to yield the linear Hansch equation and its many extended forms
Hansch (1969)	Developed the parabolic Hansch equation for dealing with extended hydrophobicity ranges
Free and Wilson (1964)	Formulated an additive model, where the activity is discretized as a simple sum of contributions from different substituents
Fujita and Ban (1971)	Simplified the Free Wilson equation estimating the activity for the non-substituted compound of the series and postulated Fujita-Ban equation that used the logarithm of activity, which brought the activity parameter in line with other free energy-related terms
Kubinyi (1976)	Investigated the transport of drugs via aqueous and lipoidal compartment systems and further refined the parabolic equation of Hansch to develop a superior bilinear (non linear) QSAR model
Hansch and Gao (1997)	Developed comparative QSAR (C-QSAR), incorporated in the C-QSAR program
Heritage and Lowis (1997)	Developed Hologram QSAR (HQSAR), where the structures are converted into all possible fragments, which are assigned specific integers, and then hashed into a fingerprint to form the molecular hologram. The bin occupancies of these holograms are used as the QSAR descriptors, encoding the chemical and topological information of molecules
Cho and workers (1998)	Developed Inverse QSAR, which helps in finding the values for the molecular descriptors that possess a desired activity/property value. In other words, it consists of finding the optimum sets of descriptor values best matching a target activity and then generating a focused library of candidate structures from the solution set of descriptor values
Labute (1999)	Developed Binary QSAR to handle binary activity measurements from high-throughput screening (e.g., pass/fail or active/inactive), and molecular descriptor vectors as input. A probability distribution for actives and inactives is then determined based on Bayes' Theorem

CLASSIFICATION OF QSAR METHODOLOGIES

Based on dimensionality: Most often the QSAR methods are categorized into following classes, based on the structural representation or the way by which the descriptor values are derived:

1D-QSAR correlating activity with global molecular properties like pKa, log *P*, *etc.*

2D-QSAR correlating activity with structural patterns like connectivity indices, 2D-pharmacophores, *etc.* without taking into account the 3D-representation of these properties

3D-QSAR correlating activity with non covalent interaction fields surrounding the molecules

4D-QSAR additionally including ensemble of ligand configurations in 3D-QSAR

5D-QSAR explicitly representing different induced-fit models in 4D-QSAR

6D-QSAR further incorporating different salvation models in 5D-QSAR

Based on the type of chemometric methods used: Sometimes QSAR methods are also classified into following two categories, depending upon the type of correlation technique employed to establish a relationship between structural properties and biological activity.

i. Linear methods including linear regression (LR), multiple linear regression (MLR), partial least-squares (PLS), and principal component analysis/regression (PCA/ PCR).

ii. Non linear methods consisting of artificial neural networks (ANN), k-nearest neighbors (kNN), and Bayesian neural nets.

LIMITATIONS OF CLASSICAL QSAR METHODOLOGIES

Classical QSAR methods are much simpler, faster and more amenable to automation than 3D-QSAR approaches. They include clearly-defined physiochemical descriptors and are best suited for the analysis of large number of compounds and computational screening of molecular databases. Though they have been used for decades to correlate and predict the activity of molecules, they suffer from serious limitations in certain situations some of which are as follows:

- Only 2D-structures considered
- Unavailability of appropriate physiochemical parameter (*e.g.* numerical descriptors for new or unusual substituents), rendering the compound unfit for inclusion in QSAR analysis
- Insufficient parameters for describing drug-receptor interactions (*e.g.* steric parameter E_s, Hammetts, *etc.*)
- Confined to only few substitutions in a common reference structure (simple variation of aromatic substituents) and works best with a congeneric series
- No representation of stereochemistry or 3D-structure of molecules, regardless of their availability
- Provide no unique solutions
- Higher risk of chance correlations
- High risk of failure due to 'too far outside' predictions
- No graphical output thereby making the interpretation of results in familiar chemical terms, frequently difficult if not impossible

- Requires considerable knowledge of substituent constants in physical organic chemistry to design a molecule, since classical QSAR equation do not directly suggest new compounds to synthesize.

PROGRESS IN 3D-QSAR APPROACHES

3D-QSAR is a broad term encompassing all those QSAR methods which correlate macroscopic target properties with computed atom-based descriptors derived from the spatial (three-dimensional) representation of the molecular structures. The methodology has emerged as a natural extension to the classical QSAR approaches pioneered by Hansch and Free-Wilson. The major drawback of 3D-QSAR techniques is that they all are based on various assumptions which are described in the subsequent section.

ASSUMPTIONS IN 3D-QSAR METHODS

None of the QSAR model can replace the experimental assays, though experimental techniques are also not free from errors. Because of many obvious problems in simulating the real world situations, not every *in vivo* parameter can be included in the QSAR modeling. However, every attempt is made to develop a model as close as possible to the real one and for this the 3D-QSAR paradigm has to rely on some basic assumptions which are given below:

- There is an underlying relationship between molecular structure and biological activity.
- Receptor binding is directly proportional to the biological activity. Differential effects on second messengers or other signaling steps which transpire between receptor binding and experimentally observed response, are not taken into consideration.
- Molecular structure can be measured and represented with a set of numbers usually called descriptors, which represent all physical, chemical and biological properties of the molecule.
- Molecules with common or related structures generally have similar physicochemical properties (the similarity principle), and thus have similar binding modes and consequently comparable biological activities. The reverse also holds true. Also, molecules located in the same region of the descriptor space present similar activity (the neighborhood principle).
- Structural properties which lead to an observed biological response are most commonly determined by the nonbonding (or noncovalent) forces, mainly steric and electrostatic.
- The observed biological effect is produced by the modeled ligand itself, and not by its metabolite or degradation product.
- The lowest energy conformation of the ligand is its bioactive conformation, and it is this single conformation of the ligand which exerts the binding effects.
- With few exceptions, the geometry of the receptor binding site is considered rigid.
- The loss of translational and rotational degrees of freedom (entropy) upon binding is believed to follow a similar pattern for all the molecules.
- Total number of rotatable bonds is the only method most frequently used to estimate the entropic cost for freezing non-terminal single-bond rotors.
- For all the modeled ligands, the protein binding site is assumed to be same.

- For all the modeled compounds, the on-off rate is supposed to be similar, i.e. the system is considered to be in equilibrium, and kinetic aspects are usually ignored.
- Some of the major factors like desolvation energetics, temperature, diffusion, transport, pH, salt concentration, *etc.* which contribute to the overall free energy of binding are difficult to handle, and thus usually ignored.
- In molecular mechanics based 3D-QSAR methods, free energy of binding is largely explained by the enthalpic component (i.e., the internal energy), which is prone to the inherent force field errors.
- Resulting QSAR model may represent one of potentially several solutions to the property–activity correlation problem.

CLASSIFICATION OF 3D-QSAR APPROACHES

3D-QSAR methods can be classified on various criteria, some of which are given in Table 5.2.

Table 5.2. Classification of 3D-QSAR approaches	
Classification	*Examples*
On the basis of intermolecular modeling, or the information used to develop QSAR	
Ligand-based 3D-QSAR	CoMFA, CoMSIA, COMPASS, GERM, CoMMA, SoMFA
Receptor-based 3D-QSAR	COMBINE, AFMoC, HIFA, CoRIA
On the basis of alignment criterion	
Alignment-dependent 3D-QSAR	CoMFA, CoMSIA, GERM, COMBINE, AFMoC, HIFA, CoRIA
Alignment-independent 3D-QSAR	COMPASS, CoMMA, HQSAR, WHIM, EVA/CoRSA, GRIND
On the basis of the chemometric technique used for correlating structural properties and activities	
Linear 3D-QSAR	CoMFA, CoMSIA, AFMoC, GERM, CoMMA, SoMFA
Non-linear 3D-QSAR	COMPASS, QPLS

CoMFA

In 1987, Cramer developed the predecessor of 3D approaches called Dynamic Lattice-Oriented Molecular Modeling System (DYLOMMS) that involves the use of PCA to extract vectors from the molecular interaction fields, which are then correlated with biological activities. Soon after this, he modified it by combining the two existing techniques - GRID and PLS, to develop a powerful 3D-QSAR methodology, Comparative Molecular Field Analysis (CoMFA). Today, CoMFA has become a proto-type of 3D-QSAR methods. A standard CoMFA procedure, as implemented in the Sybyl Software from Tripos Inc., follows the following sequential steps:

- Bioactive conformations of each molecule are determined.
- All the molecules are superimposed or aligned using either manual or automated methods, in a manner defined by the supposed mode of interaction with the receptor.

- The overlaid molecules are placed in the center of a lattice grid with a spacing of 2 Å.
- The algorithm compares, in three-dimensions, the steric and electrostatic fields calculated around the molecules with different probe groups positioned at all intersections of the lattice.
- The interaction energy or field values are correlated with the biological activity data using PLS technique, which identifies and extracts the quantitative influence of specific chemical features of molecules on their biological activity.
- The results are articulated as correlated equations with the number of latent variable terms, each of which is a linear combination of original independent lattice descriptors.
- For visual understanding, the PLS output is presented in the form of an interactive graphics consisting of colored contour plots of coefficients of the corresponding field variables at each lattice intersection, and showing the imperative favorable and unfavorable regions in three dimensional space which are considerably associated with the biological activity. Several parameters which significantly control the overall performance of the developed CoMFA model are described below; many of these are also applicable to other QSAR methodologies.

Biological Data

The popular 'GIGO' (garbage in garbage out) principle applies in every computational technique. In 3D-QSAR also, accurate activity data is determined in order to develop a good model. Though, 3D-QSAR methods can be applied to heterogeneous data sets, some below given considerations for maintaining the accuracy of biological data are necessary:

- Compounds should belong to a congeneric series (it is more important in case of classical QSAR).
- Compounds should have the same mechanism of action and same/comparable binding mode.
- The biological activities of compounds should correlate to their binding affinity and their enumerated biological responses should be measurable.
- Biological data for molecules should be obtained using uniform protocols (radioligand, activator, cofactor, pH, buffer, *etc.*) and preferably from a single source (organism/tissue/cell/protein) and single lab.
- Activity data for all the compounds should be in same units of measurement (binding/functional/IC_{50}/K_i). K_i value is preferred instead of the IC_{50} data, since it is independent of the substrate concentration.
- The ranges of biological activity covered should be as large as possible, keeping the mode of action identical. Preferably, activity range should be much larger than the standard deviations of the data; more than three logarithm units with an even spread of data is preferred.
- If possible, biological data should be symmetrically distributed around their mean, and their precision should be evenly distributed over its range of variation. If not, such skewness can be removed by log transforming the data and expressing it as $\log (1/C)$, where C refers to the molar concentration of drug producing a standard response. It is noteworthy that free energy change is proportional to the inverse log of concentration of the compound.

Compound Selection and Series Optimization

One of the major applications of QSAR is to optimize the existing leads by structural modifications so as to improve their activity and reduce/eliminate the side-effects. However, there are many issues to be taken care of while selecting substituents for the modification of compounds. Some of the important ones are given below:

- The compounds/substituents selected should be convincingly different from the existing ones, so as to minimize co-linearity among the variables.
- The chosen compounds/substituents should have the properties which behave independent of each other, thereby maximizing dissimilarity and orthogonality.
- The selection should be done in such a manner so as to map the substituent (descriptor) space with minimum number of compounds.
- Synthetic accessibility/feasibility of the selected compounds should also be taken into consideration.

Optimization of 3D-structure of the Molecules

An important issue in 3D-QSAR is how to generate and represent the starting molecular structure for analysis? The problem can be resolved both by experimental as well as computational techniques. A large number of well resolved experimentally determined crystal structures are available in databases like Cambridge Structural Database and Protein Data Bank. The crystal structures offer the advantage that some conformational information about the flexible molecule is included. However, molecular modeling methods are particularly useful for compounds that have not been made or cannot even exists under normal conditions. Computationally the 3D-structures can be generated by three methods:

- a. manually by sketching the structures interactively in a 3D-computer graphics interface or from an existing 3D-structure included in the fragment libraries,
- b. numerically by using mathematical techniques like distance geometry, quantum or molecular mechanics, and
- c. by automatic methods that are often used for building 3D-structure databases.

After the generation of starting 3D-molecular structures, their geometries are refined by minimizing their conformational energies using theoretical calculation methods. Commonly used structure optimization techniques include:

- a. molecular mechanics methods which usually does not explicitly consider the electronic motion, and thus are fast, reasonably accurate and can be used for very large molecules like enzymes,
- b. quantum mechanics or *ab initio* methods which takes into account the 3D-distribution of electrons around the nuclei, and therefore are extremely accurate but time consuming, computationally intensive and cannot handle large molecules,
- c. semi-empirical methods which are basically quantum mechanical in nature but employs an extensive use of approximations as in molecular mechanics. Generally, the molecular geometry is optimized by molecular mechanics methods, and its atomic charges are calculated mostly by semi-empirical methods or less frequently by *ab initio* methods.

Conformational Analysis of Molecules

It is a well recognized fact that each compound containing one or more single bonds exists at each moment in many different so-called *rotamers* or *conformers*. Although, small molecules may have only a single lowest energy conformation but large and flexible molecules do exists in multiple conformations at physiological conditions. Therefore, it becomes necessary to include various such conformations of the molecules in a 3D-QSAR study. Depending upon the type of molecules in the study, anyone of the following conformational search methods can be adopted:

- Systematic search (or grid search) method which generates all possible conformations, by systematically varying each of the torsion angles of a molecule by some increment, keeping the bond lengths and bond angles fixed.

- Random search method which generates a set of conformations by repetitively and randomly changing either the Cartesian (x, y, z) or the internal (bond lengths, bond angles and torsion/dihedral angles) coordinates of a starting geometry of the molecule under consideration.

- Monte Carlo method which simulates dynamic behavior of a molecule and generates the conformations by making random changes in its structure, calculating and comparing its energy with that of the previous conformation and accepting it if it is unique.

- Molecular dynamics method which employs the Newton's second law of motion (force = mass acceleration) to simulate the time-dependent movements and conformational changes in a molecular system, and results in a so-called trajectory showing how the positions and velocities of atoms in the molecular system vary with time.

- Simulated annealing which heats up the molecular system under consideration to high temperatures to overcome huge energy barriers, and after equilibrating there for sometime using molecular dynamics, cools down the system slowly and gradually to obtain the low energy conformations according to the Boltzmann distribution.

- Distance geometry algorithm which generates a random set of coordinates by selecting random distances within each pair of upper and lower bounds to form constraints in a distance matrix, which are the used to generate energetically feasible conformations of a set of molecules.

- Genetic and evolutionary algorithms which are based on the concept of biological evolution and works by first creating a population of possible solutions to the problem. The solutions with best fitness scores undergo crossovers and mutations over a time, and propagate their good characteristics down the generations to result in better solutions in the form of new conformers.

Determining Bioactive Conformations of Molecules

Bioactive conformation refers to that conformation of the molecule which gives perfect binding with the receptor. Intrinsic forces between the atoms in the molecule as well as extrinsic forces between the molecule and its surrounding environment significantly influence the bioactive conformation of the molecule. The success of any 3D-QSAR methodology depends on the determination of bioactive conformations. Bioactive conformations of the molecules can be obtained both by experimental as well as theoretical techniques. Experimental methods for establishing bioactive conformations include:

X-ray crystallography: Drug-receptor complexes generated by X-ray crystallography provide reasonably accurate information regarding 3D- structure of macromolecules.

Limitations:

- The protein needs to be crystallized and the constitution of crystallizing media is not usually similar to the physiological conditions
- The method produces a time-averaged structure, since data collection usually takes a long time
- Many times the structures are distorted due to crystal packing.
- Because of crystal instability and active-site occlusion, it is often not possible to diffuse substrates or other biologically relevant molecules into the existing crystals.
- Positions of hydrogen atoms are difficult to be resolved.
- Errors in accurately determining the structure of the ligand.

NMR spectroscopy: In this method, the 3D-structural data is obtained in solution. It is a method of choice when the molecule cannot be crystallized through experimental ways, as in case of the membrane bound receptors or receptors which have not yet been isolated due to stability, resolution or other issues. The important features of this method are:

- Since no protein crystallization is required, the conformation of the protein is not influenced by packing forces of the crystal environment
- The solution conditions (pH, ionic strength, substrate, temperature, *etc.*) can be adjusted to match the physiological conditions. The results are also highly dependent on the solvent
- Significant information regarding dynamic aspects of molecular motion can be obtained
- Takes less time but is suitable for small molecules only.
- Positions of hydrogen atoms can be resolved.
- Apolar solvents may lead to an overestimation of hydrogen bonding phenomena.
- Structure obtained from NMR may not be similar to the one obtained from experimental methods, and many times it may not represent the receptor bound conformation. Theoretically 3D-structural information can be obtained by a knowledge-based approach, called Protein/homology modeling. In this method, the primary sequence of new protein is compared with all sequences of structurally known proteins stored in a database like PDB. Proteins in the database which are found to be homologous to the unknown are retrieved and used as templates for the structural prediction of the unknown protein. However this approach is limited only to the target proteins that are amenable to structure determination. Also the quality and applicability of this method primarily depends on the sequence similarity between the protein of known structure (template) and the protein to be modeled (target).

Alignment of Molecules

One of the most crucial problems in most of the alignment-based 3D-QSAR methods is that their results are highly sensitive to the manner in which the bioactive conformations of all the molecules are superimposed over each other. In cases, where all the molecules in a data set have a common rigid core structure, molecules can be aligned easily using least-square fitting procedure. However in case of structural heterogeneity in the dataset, alignment of highly flexible molecules becomes quite difficult and time consuming.

Several approaches have been proposed to superimpose the molecules as accurately as possible, some of which are as follows:

Atom overlapping based superimposition: This method involves corresponding atom to atom pairing between the molecules. It is also called as the pharmacophore approach and is the most popular method, since it gives the best matching of the preselected atom positions. It is beneficial in identifying dissimilarity between similar molecules, but cannot be applied to molecules with different structural types where corresponding atoms are difficult to select.

Binding sites based superimposition: In this method, molecular alignment is obtained by superimposing the receptor active sites or the receptor residues that interact with the ligands. This approach is believed to be more conceivable, despite problems in conformational analysis due to enhanced degrees of freedom.

Fields/pseudofields based superimposition: This method perform superimposition by comparing the similarities in the calculated interaction energy fields between the molecules. Electrostatic similarity and molecular surface similarity indices have also been used by the researchers for molecular alignment.

Pharmacophore based superimposition: This method uses a hypothetical pharma-cophore as a useful common target template. Each molecule is conformationally directed to assume the shape obligatory for its sub-molecular features to match with either a known pharmacophore or the one which is generated during the con-formational analysis.

Multiple conformers based superimposition: This method is particularly useful in cases where the ligands may bind to a receptor in multiple ways, or when the correct binding mode is unknown and the ligands have a fair degree of conformational flexibility. For example, the 3D-QSAR method COMPASS (described in later section) iteratively determines and selects the best bioactive conformation and optimal alignment from a set of initial poses.

Calculation of Molecular Interaction Energy Fields

After superimposition, the overlaid set of molecules is positioned in the center of a lattice or grid box, to calculate interaction energies between the ligands and different probe atoms placed at each intersection of the lattice. Various aspects that are required to be taken care of while calculating the interaction energies in CoMFA methodology are as follows:

- The standard size of the grid spacing is 2 Å. The grid spacing is inversely proportional to the rigorousness of calculations. As the grid spacing decreases to 1 Å or less, the calculations becomes more intensive requiring much more computing time and disc storage space. The reduced grid spacing (0.5 Å) is usually employed while extracting interaction energy fields for a reference (most active) compound during molecular superimposition based on fields, as described earlier.
- The typical size of the grid box is 3–4 Å larger than the union surface of the overlaid molecules. Since the electrostatic/Coulombic interactions are long-range in nature, a larger grid box may be needed. Due to inherent correlation between electrostatic energies among lattice points in close proximity, a similar size grid box can be used for steric/van der Waals interactions.
- Many times the position of the grid box considerably influences the statistics particularly the number of components in the final CoMFA model. Generally, the

initial models are developed at various locations to spot the best grid position. Two approaches have been proposed to reduce the instability. The first one suggests rotating the set of overlaid molecules in a manner that they are not parallel to any of the grid edges. The second strategy recommends substituting the field value at a lattice point by average of the field values at the vertices of a cube centered on the grid point, whose side length is two-thirds of the grid spacing.

- In CoMFA, the interaction energies are calculated using probes. The probe may be a small molecule like water, or a chemical fragment such as a methyl group. The electrostatic energies are calculated with H^+ probe, whereas a sp_3 hybridized carbon atom with an effective radius of 1.53 Å and a +1.0 charge is used as probe for including the steric energies. Each probe is positioned in turn at every intersection point of the lattice, and the interaction energies between the probe and each of the compounds are calculated using different molecular force fields.

- A force field is a mathematical equation, which using a combination of bond lengths, bond angles, dihedral angles, interatomic distances along with coordinates and other parameters, empirically fit the potential energy surface. Major forces encountered in the drug-receptor intermolecular interactions include electrostatic/ Coulombic, hydrogen bonding, steric/van der Waals and hydrophobic. The electrostatic and hydrogen bonding interactions are responsible for ligand-receptor specificity, whereas hydrophobic interactions generally provide the strength for binding. The most commonly employed fields in CoMFA are steric and electrostatic, which are mainly enthalpic in nature. However, many times the entropic effects, in the form of hydrophobic interactions, are also included in the CoMFA analysis. Creativity of the research and the validity of the underlying theory are the major parameters deciding the type of field to be generated and included in a CoMFA model.

- In CoMFA, the standard Lennard-Jones function is used to model the van der Waals interactions whereas electrostatic interactions are determined by the Coulomb's law. The slope of the Lennard-Jones potentials is very steep close to the van der Waals surface, as a result of which the potential energy at lattice points in the proximity of the surface changes significantly. This implies that a trivial difference in the mutual shift or conformational changes of the compounds may result in very large differences in energy values. Moreover, the Lennard-Jones and Coulombic potentials show singularities (unacceptably large values) at the atomic positions. Therefore to avoid all these problems in CoMFA, the cut-off values (± 30 kcal/mol) for steric and electrostatic energy are defined.

Data Pretreatment and Scaling

Before performing the actual chemometric analysis in 3D-QSAR, the raw data is usually pretreated to minimize redundancy (chances of repetition). One of the common reduction methods is based on the standard deviation cut-off, in which all the energy columns with a low standard deviation are eliminated from the data, since they require longer computing time without contributing significantly to the results. Similarly several variable selection methods are available, which can be used to reduce collinearity among the descriptors thereby preventing data over-fitting and improving the prediction performance of the model. Also, in CoMFA, the steric and electrostatic values are amended by using cut-offs (± 30 kcal/mol, as mentioned earlier), depending upon the position of the lattice point. Many times after pretreatment, the data is subjected to scaling which assigns equal weight to all the descriptors and places them on a common platform for a meaningful statistical analysis. Scaling significantly improves the signal to noise ratio and also allows ranking the relative importance of individual variables. Different scaling techniques are available and can be used effectively in 3D-QSAR approaches. For example: autoscaling scales the variables to zero mean and a unit standard deviation by dividing each column with its standard deviation, block-scaling provides each category of variables with the same weight by dividing the initial autoscaling weights of descriptors in one class by the square root of the number of descriptors in that class (CoMFA standard scaling), and block-adjusted scaling which is particularly useful when other variables are included along with the energy values in the analysis. This scaling gives other variables a comparable weight to the total variables. Sometimes the pretreated data is subjected to centering by subtracting the column means from all the data. This does not change any coefficient values or comparative weights of the descriptors, but the number of significant components from PLS may be one less than from the data without centering. The method is supposed to improve the ease of interpretation and numerical stability.

Model Generation and its Validation

After pretreatment and scaling of the descriptors (interaction energies and other variables, if necessary), they are correlated to the biological activities of the molecules, assuming a linear relationship between them . Since the number of independent (x) variables in CoMFA is much larger than the number of compounds in the data set, the traditional linear regression analysis cannot be used to perform the fitting process. Therefore to extract a stable and best QSAR model from a range of possible solutions, the partial least-squares (PLS) technique is used. Other methods to model linear relationships include MLR, PCA, PCR, *etc.* However many times the relationship between the dependent (y) and independent (x) variables is not linear or it can't be predicted, in such cases non-linear chemometric methods like neural networks are employed; these methods make no assumption about the relationship between the variables during training and model development. Most of these chemometric techniques for QSAR modeling are discussed in the later sections. The most important criterion for judging the quality of a QSAR model is its ability to predict accurately not only the activities of molecules that form part of training set (internal prediction), but also of molecules not included in the development of the model (external prediction). The internal predictive capability of the model can be judged from cross-validated by techniques like leave-one-out and leave-group-out, whereas its external predictivity can be evaluated by using a separate set of molecules (the test set) not included in the model development. To further assess the robustness and statistical confidence of the derived models Fischer statistics, randomization (y-scrambling) and bootstrapping analysis are also performed. All these cross validation methods have been explained in the later sections.

Display of Results

CoMFA generates an equation correlating the biological activity with the contribution of interaction energy fields at every grid point. To allow simple and easy visual interpretation, results are generally shown as coefficient (or scalar product of coefficients and standard deviation) contour plots, depicting important regions in space around the molecules where specific structural modifications significantly alters the activity. Generally, two types of contours are shown for each interaction energy field: the positive and negative contours. The contours for steric fields are shown in green (positive contours, more bulk favored) and yellow (negative contours, less bulk favored), while the electrostatic field contours are displayed in red (positive contours, electronegative substituents favored) and blue (negative contours, electropositive substituents favored) colors. In addition of contour plots, CoMFA also provides two types of plots from PLS models: score plots and loading/weight plots. Score plots between biological activity (Y-scores) and latent variables (X-scores) show relationship between the activity and the structures, whereas plots of latent variables (X-scores) display the similarity/dissimilarity between the molecules, and their clustering propensities.

DRAWBACKS AND LIMITATIONS OF CoMFA

Despite of offering many advantages over classical QSAR and good performance in various practical applications, CoMFA has several pitfalls and imperfections as given below:

- Since the time of its origin in 1988, numerous applications of the CoMFA method in different fields have been published. Several data sets have been investigated; the first being the binding affinity of the steroid data set for human corticosteroid-binding globulins (CBG) and testosterone-binding globulins (TBG). Many successful endeavors of CoMFA approach in the areas of enzyme highly sensitive to bioactive conformation, different binding modes of ligands, alignment rules and number of components
- Too many adjustable parameters like overall orientation, lattice placement, step size, probe atom type, *etc.*
- Uncertainty in selection of compounds and variables
- Fragmented contour maps with variable selection procedures
- Hydrophobicity not well-quantified
- Cut-off limits used
- Low signal to noise ratio due to many useless field variables
- Imperfections in potential energy functions
- Various practical problems with PLS
- Applicable only to *in vitro* data

Since the time of its origin in 1988, numerous applications of the CoMFA method in different fields have been published. Several data sets have been investigated; the first being the binding affinity of the steroid data set for human corticosteroid-binding globulins (CBG) and testosterone-binding globulins (TBG). Many successful endeavors of CoMFA approach in the areas of enzyme inhibition, agrochemistry (pesticides, insecticides or herbicides), physicochemistry (partition coefficients, capacity factors, enantio-separation factors and 13C chemical shifts), ADME and toxicity, thermodynamics and kinetics have also been exhaustively appraised in several reviews.

MSA

Molecular Shape Analysis (MSA) is a ligand-based 3D-QSAR formalism (strict adherence) which attempts to merge conformational analysis with the classical Hansch approach. It deals with the quantitative characterization, representation and manipulation of molecular shape in the construction of a QSAR model. The methodology begins by subjecting each molecule in the data set to a fixed valence geometry intramolecular conformational analysis with a scan at 30° increments for all torsion angles except for amide N(C=O) torsion which is scanned at 180° increment. The conformational energies are estimated using a fixed valence geometry molecular mechanics force-field consisting of a dispersion/steric, electrostatic, and, if applicable, hydrogen bonding contributions. For each compound, all apparent intramolecular energy minima are identified and recorded, each of which are then used as starting points in rigorous fixed valence geometry energy minimizations. Both apparently as well as rigorously minimized energy conformations are aspirants for the 'active' conformation of each analog in the ensuing steps. To identify the active conformation of each analog, the LBA-LCS (loss in biological activity-loss in conformational stability) approach is used; this is based on the identification of stable low-energy intramolecular conformer states common to the active analogs, which is a high energy, unstable state for the inactive analogs. A shape reference structure is selected as the mutant shape generated by the common and difference volume combinations realized by multiple compound alignments or active conformations. The potential active conformation of each compound in the data set is pair-wise compared and aligned with the shape reference. This is followed by the calculation of various descriptors which measure relative molecular shape similarity. One of the important shape variables is the common overlap steric volume (COSV) between pairs of molecules as a function of conformation and relative intermolecular geometry. It actually measures how much steric space a pair of molecules share under a prescribed intermolecular relationship. Two other descriptors are also arbitrarily defined as alternate mathematical representations of COSV that can advantageously be used in developing empirical QSARs; one has the dimensions of area but is not a physical measure of common atomic surface areas between two molecules, and another has the dimensions of length but is not a cumulative measure of distances between the molecules. These pair-wise shape variables can also be amalgamated with the non-shape thermodynamic and electronic descriptors including the terms from the Hansch equation (E_s) in developing a MSA 3DQSAR model. The shape similarity descriptors along with the non-shape variables are eventually correlated with the biological activities of the molecules using the MLR technique, however, other chemometric methods like PLS and GA can also be employed. The MSA results can be graphically represented as a picture of the most active analog placed in its active conformation or as the superimposition of shape descriptors onto the molecular geometry of the most active molecule. Some of the recent successful applications of MSA include the generation of useful 3D-QSAR models of the allosteric modulators of muscarinic receptors, anticoccidial triazines, cholecystokinin-A receptor antagonists, and indanone-benzylpiperidine inhibitors of acetylcholinesterase . MSA is being provided in the Cerius2 software from Accelrys Inc.

GRID

GRID was the first tailor-made program designed for the medicinal chemist as an alternative to the original CoMFA approach. It calculates the interaction energy fields in molecular field analysis and determines the energetically favorable binding sites on molecules of known structure. Though the approach is similar to CoMFA in that it too computes explicit non-bonded (or non-covalent) interactions between a molecule of known three-dimensional structure and a probe (i.e. a small chemical group with user-defined properties) located at the sample positions on a lattice throughout and around the macromolecule, it offers two distinct advantages; first is the use of a 6-4 potential function for calculating the interaction energies, which is smoother than the 6–12 form of the Lennard-Jones type in CoMFA, and second is, the availability of different types of probes. The program in addition of computing the regular steric and electrostatic potentials, also calculates the hydrogen bonding potential using a hydrogen bond donor and acceptor, and the hydrophobic potential using a "DRY probe". Later on a water probe was added to calculate hydrophobic interactions. Since the water probe is not only electrically neutral but can also donate and accept a hydrogen bond, the energies determined using this probe are supposed to embrace steric and hydrogen bonding interactions also, besides representing the hydrophobic interaction energy like log P due to its molecular surface area. In addition to the water and DRY probes, other probes which are usually used singly, include the methyl group, the amine NH_2 group, the carboxylate group and the hydroxyl group. Contour surfaces are calculated at various energy levels for each probe for every point on the grid and are displayed graphically along with the protein structure. While negative energy levels of the contours describe regions at which ligand binding should be favored, positive energy levels normally characterize the shape of the target. Some of the recent applications of the GRID method include determining energetically favorable binding sites and characterization of their surface properties, building predictive pharmacophore models, classification and comparison of ligand-binding sites, and rational design of potent inhibitors of influenza virus sialidase. Many times GRID maps are also used as input descriptors in CoMFA, GOLPE or SIMCA for QSAR or 3D-QSAR analyses. It is possible to use these interaction energies in a statistical technique to relate to the biological activity in a quantitative manner. The GRID software is supplied by Molecular Discovery Ltd.

HASL

The Hypothetical Active Site Lattice (HASL) method is an inverse grid-based approach which represents the shapes of the molecules inside an active site as a collection of grid points. The methodology begins with the intermediate conversion of the Cartesian coordinates (x, y, z) of a superposed set of molecules to a 3D-grid consisting of the regularly-spaced points that are:

- arranged orthogonally to each other
- separated by a particular distance termed as the resolution (which determines the number of grid points representing a molecule)
- all sprawl within the van der Waals radii of the atoms constituting the molecule

The resulting framework of points is referred to as the molecular lattice and represents the receptor active site map. The overall lattice dimensions are dependent on the size of the molecules and the resolution chosen. Typically, a reference molecule is selected arbitrarily and its user-defined conformations similar in shape and that have been energy-minimized, are used to generate the HASL. The selected conformation of the reference molecule is centered about the origin of a Cartesian coordinate system, and a regular grid with a chosen resolution is then laid over the molecule. All grid points lying within the van der Waals radii of the atoms of the molecule are designated as 'occupied' and form the molecular lattice. The electronic properties of the occupying atoms are distinctly represented by assigning the lattice points a 'HASL-type' value based on the electron density of the atoms, which constitute the fourth dimension of the molecular lattice. The values of +1, −1 and 0 are assigned to the electron-rich (e.g. O, N), electron-poor (e.g. C in C=O) and neutral atoms/substituents, which roughly represent H-bond acceptors, donors, and lipophilic atom types, respectively. Such internal atom type designations allow apparently different structures to be overlaid with an equivalent electronic "sense", (i.e. similar atomic characteristics of two molecules can be superimposed in 3D space), to obtain a maximum complementarity of space and physiochemical character within that space. Similar to electron density, other user-selected physio-chemical properties such as hydrophobicity, can also be employed as the fourth dimension. A second molecule is subsequently selected and subjected to the same routine, generating its 4D lattice which is then compared and consequently aligned to that of the stationary reference molecule. In order to optimally align the molecules based on their lattices, a systematic search is performed which involves a stepped progression of translational and rotational movements, with an intermediate lattice generated at each step, until a perfect match is obtained. The extent of similarity between the two molecules is calculated according to a fitting function, based upon the degree of correspondence between the points of the two lattices, i.e, on the number of points the two lattices have in common. Once the best possible alignment between the two molecular lattices is obtained, those lattice points of the fitted molecule which are not yet in common with the reference molecule are added to create a new composite construct or larger reference lattice containing the information from both the molecules. This fitting and merging process is then repeated to include all the molecules of the training set in the growing HASL, resulting in a reference lattice entailing every point from all the molecular lattices. In order to determine the activity contributions from different lattice points, initially the experimental activity value of a molecule is homogeneously divided among its all lattice points. For lattice points which are shared by more than one molecule, the partial bioactivity values are, at first, averaged over these points and, afterwards adjusted by an iterative protocol to fit the experimental activity data of the entire training set. This iteratively optimized HASL is then used as a standardized model to predict the activities of untested molecules. The bioactivity of a specific compound is forecasted by summing all the partial activity values at points in common with the composite reference lattice. Some of the successful applications of HASL approach include the analysis of the in vitro antimalarial activity of artemisinin analogs, in vitro biochemical and in vivo gastric antisecretory activity of substituted imidazo[1,2-α]pyridines, sequence specificity of DNA alkylation by uracil mustard, and the generation of putative pharmacophoric models of the HIV-1 protease inhibitors. HASL is a copyrighted program of Hypothesis Software and eduSofLC, and also comes as one of the modules in Sybyl Software.

CoMSIA

Comparative Molecular Similarity Indices Analysis (CoMSIA) was developed to overcome certain limitations of CoMFA. In CoMSIA, molecular similarity indices calculated from modified SEAL similarity fields are employed as descriptors to simultaneously consider steric, electrostatic, hydrophobic and hydrogen bonding properties. These indices are estimated indirectly by comparing the similarity of each molecule in the dataset with a common probe atom (having a radius of 1 Å, charge of +1 and hydrophobicity of +1) positioned at the intersections of a surrounding grid/lattice. For computing similarity at all grid points, the mutual distances between the probe atom and the atoms of the molecules in the aligned dataset are also taken into account. To describe this distance-dependence and calculate the molecular properties, Gaussian-type functions are employed. Since the underlying Gaussian-type functional forms are 'smooth' with no singularities, their slopes are not as steep as the Coulombic and Lennard-Jones potentials in CoMFA; therefore, no arbitrary cut-off limits are required to be defined. These functions tend to produce values within a reasonable range, even in the case of overlapping atoms. Despite the fact that CoMSIA also suffer from most of the limitations of CoMFA, it offers following distinctive advantages:-

- Use of the Gaussian distribution of similarity indices, which avoids the abrupt changes in grid-based probe–atom interactions
- The choice of similarity probe, is not limited to either steric or electrostatic potential fields but also include hydrophobic and hydrogen bonding (hydrogen bond acceptors and donors) fields
- Effect of the solvent entropic terms can also be included by using a hydrophobic probe
- The standard CoMFA contours highlights those regions in space where the aligned molecules would favorably or unfavorably interact with a possible receptor environment. On the other hand, the CoMSIA contours indicate those areas within the region occupied by the ligands that "favor" or "dislike" the presence of a group with a particular physicochemical property. This relationship between the required properties and a probable ligand shape is a more direct guide to substantiate whether all features imperative for activity are present in the structures being considered. Some of the recent applications of CoMSIA include generation of predictive 3D-QSAR models of boron-containing dipeptides as proteasome inhibitors, hydroxamic acid derivatives as urease inhibitors, thiazolidin-4-one derivatives as anti-HIV-1 agents, and thiazolidinediones derivatives as aldose reductase inhibitors . CoMSIA is provided by Tripos Inc. in the Sybyl software, along with CoMFA.

GERM

Genetically Evolved Receptor Models (GERM) is a technique for 3D QSAR and for constructing useful three dimensional models of macromolecular binding sites in the absence of a crystallographically-determined or homology modeled structure of the target receptor. The primary requirement for GERM is a structure–activity series for which a sensible alignment of realistic conformers has been determined. The methodology consists of enclosing the superimposed set of molecules in a shell of atoms (analogous to the first layer of atoms in the active site) and allocating these atoms with explicit atom types (aliphatic H, polar H, *etc.* to match the types of atoms usually found in the proteins). Aliphatic carbon atoms are disseminated uniformly over a sphere surrounding the training set of aligned ligands, and their positions are adjusted to obtain maximum van der Waals interaction between the model carbon atoms and the ligand molecules. Once the positions of the carbons have been recognized, they can be occupied by any of the atom types, including no atom at all. One practical problem arises when the number of shell atoms and their atom types increases, since the number of possible combinations rises to a huge value thereby rendering it impossible to systematically find a best possible model. The method therefore makes use of the genetic algorithms (GA) to solve this highly multi-dimensional search problem. The ligands in the training set are then docked into a GA generated receptor active site model, one at a time, and the intermolecular nonbonded interaction energies (van der Waals and electrostatic terms) are computed using a CHARMm molecular mechanics force field. Finally these calculated interaction energies are correlated with the biological activities of the molecules. The affirmative feature of this method is that the model is presented as a 3D-display of the receptor properties in space. The limitation of GERM methodology is that it considers only a single conformation of each ligand in the training set, as well as its single orientation in the binding site. Since this method is based on the computation of interaction energies with the hypothetical receptor, it is subjected to all the limitations of such methods including the alignment problem. However, if all the molecules of the set do bind in a manner that doesn't alter the binding site too much; GERM could be a good approach. The method has been applied profitably on a series of sweeteners, correlating their bioactivities with the calculated intermolecular energy. The methodology has a fair potential for application in screening 3D-structural databases to find new leads, or in combination with de novo ligand-design programs [the program GERM is available from D. Eric Walters, Associate Professor, Finch University of Health Sciences, North Chicago, USA].

COMBINE

Comparative Binding Energy Analysis (COMBINE) method was developed to take advantage of the structural data from ligand-macromolecule complexes, in a 3D-QSAR paradigm. The technique is based upon the hypothesis that the free energy of binding can be correlated with a subset of energy components calculated from the structures of receptors and ligands in bound and unbound forms. The ligands are divided into fragments and the same number of fragments is allocated to all the compounds, adding "dummy" fragments to the ligands lacking a particular fragment. The non-bonded (van der Waals and electrostatic) interaction energies are computed between each residue of the receptor and every fragment of the ligand, using a molecular mechanics force field. The energies are also calculated between all pairs of residues/fragments for the complexes and for the free ligands and receptor. The electrostatic interactions are computed using a distance-dependent dielectric constant, and no cutoff limits are employed for the non-bonded interactions. The insignificant descriptors are then eliminated from the data using the variable selection utility in GOLPE program, and finally the biological activities of the molecules are correlated with the interaction energy values by employing PLS technique. Like all other interaction energy based 3D-QSAR approaches, COMBINE also suffers from the inherent errors involved in the computation of these energies. Also, the predictive ability of the method can be enhanced by making improvements in various aspects like the description of the electrostatic term, the inclusion of suitable descriptors for solvation and entropic effects, and the optimization of particular facets of the methodology, such as the choice of ligand fragment definitions and the details of the variable selection protocol. Recently COMBINE methodology has been utilized to build 3D-QSAR models to determine the selectivity and specificity of Ras proteins, predict binding affinity of nonpeptide inhibitors of HIV-1 protease, and to identify amino acid residues in haloalkane dehalogenase LinB that modulate its substrate specificity.

CoMMA

Comparative Molecular Moment Analysis (CoMMA) is one of the unique alignment-independent 3D QSAR techniques, which involves the computation of descriptors based molecular similarity on the spatial moments of molecular mass (shape) and charge distributions up to and including second order as well as related quantities. With respect to each molecular structure, two Cartesian reference frames are then defined. One frame is the principal inertial axes calculated with respect to the center-of-mass. For neutral molecular species, the other reference frame is the principal quadrupolar axes calculated with respect to the molecular "center-of-dipole". Dipolar, quadrupolar, and displacement descriptors are then calculated with reference to the principal inertial axes translated such that its origin is superposed on the center-of-dipole. It is noteworthy that these descriptors are obtained after translation to the center of mass as well as the center of dipole for each molecule, to keep the system alignment-independent. Finally these molecular moment descriptors are correlated with the biological activities of molecules using the PLS technique. Literature reports suggest that CoMMA descriptors are sensitive to molecular conformations, but less sensitive than CoMFA field parameters. The authors propose that the CoMMA descriptors have a potential role in addressing the issues like large scale screening and molecular diversity. The method has been used to build robust 3D-QSAR models to comprehend the structure-activity relationships of the benchmark steroid data set, and to develop combinatorial QSAR of ambergris fragrance compounds. A web version of the CoMMA program is provided by the IBM informatics group.

CoMSA

Comparative Molecular Surface Analysis (CoMSA) is a non-grid 3D-QSAR approach. It involves the use of the molecular surface for defining those regions of the compounds which are required to be compared using the mean electrostatic potentials. The methodology proceeds by subjecting the molecules in the data set to geometry optimization and assigning them with partial atomic charges. The Kohonen's self-organizing maps (SOM, a type of neural network) are then employed to transform the three dimensional surface of the molecules into two-dimensional topographical maps, by extracting the signals from the Cartesian coordinates of the points sampled randomly at the van der Waals surface of the molecules. The partial atomic charges of the atomic molecular representations are also projected onto the 2D-topographical maps. The molecular electrostatic potentials (MEPs) are calculated at the surface points and a mean value of the potential analogous to the respective points found in each grid cell (CoMFA like methods) is utilized to explain this cell. The calculated mean electrostatic potential values are converted into vectors and the vectors expressing all the molecules in the series are superimposed onto a matrix, by comparing the respective topographical maps of the molecules. The ensuing comparative matrix of the mean electrostatic potentials (transformed into vectors) is finally used to develop a 3D-QSAR model using the PLS technique. The distinctive feature of CoMSA is that, in contrast to CoMFA and related approaches, it compares the molecular properties explaining not a discrete set of points but the mean electrostatic potential values (MEPs) calculated for a certain area of the molecular surface. Recently a receptor-dependent CoMSA model, using multipose molecular docking and iterative variable elimination PLS (IVE-PLS), has been developed and applied on sulforaphane compounds as activators of quinone reductase. Other recent applications of CoMSA include the modeling of pKa values of benzoic acids, and hypolipidemic asarones, virtual combinatorial library screening of styryl quinoline HIV 1 blocking agents, and determination of the binding mode for a series of benzoxazine oxytocin antagonists using docking and 3D-QSAR studies.

AFMoC

Adaptation of Fields for Molecular Comparison (AFMoC) is a 3D-QSAR method involving fields derived from the protein environments (and not from the superimposed ligands as in CoMFA), therefore it is also known as a 'reverse' CoMFA (=AFMoC) approach. The methodology begins by placing a regularly-spaced grid into the receptor binding site, followed by mapping of the knowledge based pair-potentials between protein atoms and ligand atom probes onto the grid intersections resulting in the potential fields. Based on these potential fields, interaction fields are generated by multiplying distance-dependent atom-type properties of actual ligands docked into the active site with the neighboring grid values. These atom-type specific interaction fields are then correlated with the binding affinities of the molecules using PLS technique, which assigns individual weighting factors to each field value. Finally, the results are displayed graphically by using contribution maps, and binding affinities of novel ligands are predicted by applying the derived 3D-QSAR equation. The distinctive features of this approach include:

- A tailor-made scoring function is combined with a protein-based CoMFA approach, thereby overcoming the prerequisite to involve complete ligand training sets
- The gradual shift from generally valid knowledge-based potentials to protein-specific pair-potentials, reflects the amount and the degree of structural diversity existing in the ligand training data
- Atom-type specific interaction fields are used which are mutually orthogonal in nature and thus eases the interpretation of PLS results
- In addition of the enthalpic contribution, the methodology is also expected to include the entropic effects resulting from (de-)solvation, since structural knowledge from experimentally determined complexes is converted into statistical pair potentials. Some of the thriving applications of AFMoC include building predictive 3D-QSAR models for 1-deoxyxylulose-5-phosphate (DOXP)-reductoisomerase inhibitors, 3-oxybenzamides as potent inhibitors of the coagulation protease factor Xa, thermolysin and glycogen phosphorylase b inhibitors, and for analyzing selectivity- and affinity-determining features of carbonic anhydrase isozymes . Recently the methodology has been modified to account for the multiple ligand conformations in an ensemble of protein configurations. The improved method has been termed as consensus AFMoC (AFMoC), and was validated on the thrombin inhibitors.

CoRIA AND ITS VARIANTS

Comparative Residue Interaction Analysis (CoRIA) is a 3D-QSAR approach which uses the descriptors that describe the thermodynamic events involved in ligand binding, to explore both the qualitative as well as the quantitative facets of the ligand–receptor recognition process. Initial CoRIA methodology simply consisted of calculating the non-bonded (van der Waals and Coulombic) interaction energies between the ligand and the individual active site residues of the receptor that are involved in interaction with the ligand. Employing the genetic version of PLS technique (G/PLS), these energies were then correlated with the biological activities of molecules, along with the other physiochemical variables describing the thermodynamics of binding like, lipophilicity, molar refractivity, surface area, molecular volume, strain energy, *etc.* Later on to deal with the problems of peptide QSAR, this approach was further extended and modified to develop two new variants of CoRIA: reverse-CoRIA (rCoRIA) and mixed-CoRIA (mCoRIA). In these methodologies, the peptide (ligand) is fragmented into individual amino acids and the interaction energies (van der Waals, Coulombic and hydrophobic interactions) of each amino acid in the peptide with the receptor as a whole (rCoRIA) and with individual active site residues in the receptor (mCoRIA) are calculated, which along with other thermodynamic descriptors (like free energy of solvation, entropy loss on binding, strain energy, and solvent assessable surface area) are used as independent variables that are correlated to the biological activity by G/PLS chemometric method. CoRIA methodologies makes complete use of the wealth of knowledge contained in the ligand-receptor complexes and extract crucial information regarding the nature and type of important interactions at the level of both the receptor and the ligand, which can be directly employed in the design of new molecules and receptors. The approaches have the ability to forecast modifications in both the ligand as well as the receptor, provided structures of some ligand–receptor complexes are available. The methodology has been successfully applied to study the interactions of inhibitors with Cyclooxygenase-2, MurF Enzyme of Strepto-coccus pneumonia, HIV-1 integrase, and peptides binding to MHC class-I molecule HLA-A*0201. However, these methods are difficult to be applied on small organic molecules, because unlike peptides there is no logical or universally accepted protocol for fragmenting small molecules. Also the methodologies can be further improved by solvating entire ligand-protein complexes, extensive conformational sampling by molecular dynamics, inclusion of other important interactions like hydrogen bonding, *etc.*

OTHER 3D-QSAR METHODOLOGIES

In addition of the above mentioned formalisms, several other 3D-QSAR methodologies have been developed. Some of them are as follows:

Method: Compass

Steps

- Conformational analysis is carried out to determine the probable bioactive conformation of each ligand
- descriptors measuring surface shape or polar functionality of each ligand's pose in a specific alignment in the vicinity of a particular point in space are then computed
- a neural network is constructed and models built, realignment of molecules is continuously carried out to achieve the best fit to the binding site with improvements in the neural network model
- the final model is developed from these improved and realigned molecular poses

Method: RSA/RSM/CoRSA (Receptor Surface Analysis/Modeling, Comparative Receptor Surface Analysis)

Steps

- The structures of molecules are optimized and superimposed in their bioactive conformation
- a receptor–complementary surface is generated using shape fields (defined by some distance–dependent function) that encloses a volume common to all the aligned molecules and which represents their aggregate molecular shape
- the putative chemical properties of the receptor at every surface point are computed

- PLS models are developed that correlate surface properties with molecular activities

Method: VFA (Voronoi Field Analysis)

Steps

- A conformational analysis, minimization and superimposition of all the molecules is first carried out.
- the volume occupied by superimposed set of molecules is divided into subspaces referred to as Voronoi polyhedral, each including a reference point (an atom) with certain coordinates as explained in the following steps
- first a template (the simplest) molecule is selected and all the atoms of the template molecule are allocated as initial reference points
- next the largest molecule in the dataset is superimposed on the template in terms of the number of atoms and new reference points are designated if this point is greater than 1 Å distance of the reference points identified in the above step.
- the above two steps are repeated with superimposition of other molecules in decreasing order of their size, each time defining isolated atoms as new reference points by the criteria stated above, until all compounds are superimposed
- a cuboid with six tangential planes divided into a 3D-lattice with a spacing of 0.3Å, surrounding the union volume of the superposed set of molecules is constructed. This gives the Voronoi polyhedral.
- the potential and electrostatic energy indices at each lattice point is computed according to the 'hard-sphere potential' model and Coulomb's law respectively
- the PLS algorithm is then applied to correlate independent steric and electrostatic latent variables with the activity index.

Method: PARM (Pseudo Atomic Receptor Model)

Steps

- fifteen types of pseudo receptor atoms types possibly found in a protein are selected
- the molecules are superimposed and a 3D-grid around their common surface is generated
- pre-defined atom types and formal charge at these grid points are assigned using a genetic algorithm; this is based on the charge of the ligand atom closest to the grid point
- a GA-based initial population of individuals or receptor models are generated
- van der Waals and electrostatic interaction energies between each ligand and the receptor model are computed and are correlated to their molecular activities using a linear regression technique.

Method: SOMFA (Self Organizing Molecular Field Analysis)

Steps

- Firstly the mean activity of training set is subtracted from the activity of each molecule to obtain their mean centered activity values
- a 3D-grid around the molecules with values at the grid points signifying the shape or electrostatic potential is generated
- the shape or electrostatic potential value at every grid point for each molecule is multiplied by its mean centered activity

- the grid values for each molecule are summed up to give the master grids for each property
- the so called SOMFA property/ descriptors from the master grid values are then calculated and correlated with the logtransformed molecular activities

Method: FLUFF-BALL

Steps

- A semiautomatic superimposition of the molecules based on a novel field-fitting procedure called Flexible Ligand Unified Force Field (FLUFF) is carried out; this is a MMFF94 force field that is customized to impart flexibility to the ligand to maximize adaptation/similarity between the steric and electrostatic field volumes of the ligand and the template
- the internal coordinate system is attached to the template molecule by placing the vertices of the local grid at the atomic centers of the template, using the Boundless Adaptive Localized Ligand (BALL) approach, thus rendering the system gridindependent
- the similarity between ligands and template is evaluated, and the computed steric and electrostatic descriptors are correlated with the biological activities using the PLS technique.

Method: CoMASA (Comparative Molecular Active Site Analysis)

Steps

- The molecules are first superimposed and their interatomic distances calculated
- then is extracted the co-ordinates of the molecular representation (instead of the lattice points as in CoMFA) by continuously removing the atoms that are closer to each other, and replacing them with pseudo atoms (created from their weighted average), until the distances between all the atoms/pseudo atoms are greater than the threshold value of 0.75 Å
- the interaction energies (steric, electrostatic and hydrophobic properties) are then computed for each molecule at these points by different evaluation functions and finally these are correlated with their molecular activities using PLS.

Method: CoMPIA (Comparative Molecule/Pseudoreceptor Interaction Analysis)

Steps

- The geometry of the molecules is optimized which is followed by their superimposition based on a common template molecule
- the resulting space encompassed by the set of superimposed molecules is partitioned into grids with sufficient number of lattice points to accommodate all the probe atoms
- nine different types of hybrid atoms/probes are distributed at each lattice point using a genetic algorithm
- the steric, electrostatic and hydrophobic interactions between different probes and every molecule in the set are computed and then correlated with the biological activities using PLS

STATISTICAL METHODS USED FOR BUILDING QSAR MODELS

Statistical or chemometric techniques form the mathematical foundation for building a QSAR model. Some of these methods are briefly described in Table 5.3.

Table 5.3: Statistical techniques for building QSAR models
Linear Regression Analysis (RA)
Simple linear regression
Multiple linear regression (MLR)
Stepwise multiple linear regression
Multivariate data analysis
Principal component analysis (PCA)
Principal components regression (PCR)
Partial least square analysis (PLS)
Genetic function approximation (GFA)
Genetic partial least squares (G/PLS)
Pattern recognition
Cluster analysis
Artificial neural networks (ANNs)
k-nearest neighbor (*k*NN)

Among the increasing pool of various statistical methods available in the literature, Linear Regression analyses are considered as an easily interpretable methods indicated for QSAR analysis. These regression techniques construct a statistical model to represent the correlation of one or more independent variables (x) with a dependent explicative variable (y). The model can be utilized to predict y from the knowledge of x variables, which can be either quantitative or qualitative. Simple linear regression, multiple linear regression, and stepwise multiple linear regression are some of its variants. Simple linear regression method performs a standard linear regression calculation to generate a set of QSAR equations that include a single independent descriptor x and a dependent variable y. Thus, a one-term linear equation is produced separately for each independent variable from the descriptor set. This technique is suitable for gene rating simple relationships between structure and activity exploring some of the most important descriptors governing the activity. However, the interaction of multiple descriptors is ignored. The simple linear regression can be expressed by the equation:

$$y = a + bx$$

where the dependent variable y is expressed in terms of the independent variable x by means of two parameters: the constant a, also referred to as the intercept and the regression coefficient b. **Multiple linear regression (MLR)** also referred to as the linear free-energy relationship (LFER) method, is an extension of the simple regression analysis to more than one dimension. MLR generates QSAR equations by performing standard multivariable regression calculations to identify the dependence of a drug property on any or all of the descriptors under investigation. The possibility of chance correlation is checked through the values of multiple correlation coefficient (r), Student's t-value; Fisher's F ratio, standard deviation (s), and through independent tests like the leave-one-out (LOO) method. The significance of correlation can be judged through cross-validated correlation coefficient (r_{cv}^2 or q^2) values and also by the y-scrambling technique. MLR assumes that all variable are independent, and not correlated. However, in the multivariate case, i.e. MLR analysis involving more than one independent variable, the relationship is expressed with the following single multiple term linear equation:

$$y = b_0 + b_1 x_1 + b_2 x_2 + \ldots + b_m x_m + e$$

the MLR analysis estimates the regression coefficients (b_i), by minimizing the residual error (e), which quantify the deviation of a particular point from the regression line, as in the case of simple linear regression.

Stepwise multiple linear regression is a commonly used variant of MLR which also creates a multiple-term linear equation, but not all the independent variables are used. In contrast to MLR, each independent variable is sequentially added to the equation and new regression is performed every time. The new term is preserved only if the model passes a test for significance. This regression technique is especially useful when the number of descriptors is large and the key descriptors are unknown. The methods described above have now been replaced by *multivariate chemometric methods* which try to explain an extended set of variables by means of a reduced number of new latent variables possessing the maximum amount of information relevant to the problem. These techniques project multivariate data into a space of lower dimensions providing insight to visualize, classify, and model large data sets. These latent variables are orthogonal and hence can be used in multiple linear regressions.

Partial least squares (PLS) is an iterative regression procedure that produces its solutions based on linear transformation of a large number of original descriptors to a small number of new orthogonal terms called latent variables. PLS gives a statistically robust solution even when the independent variables are highly interrelated among themselves, or when the independent variables exceed the number of observations. Thus, PLS is able to analyze complex structure-activity data in a more realistic way, and effectively interpret the influence of molecular structure on biological activity. This is one of the standard statistical methods used for the development of predictive 3D-QSAR models.

Principal components analysis (PCA) is another data reduction technique that does not generate a QSAR model but seeks for relationships among independent variables. It then creates a new set of orthogonal descriptors - referred to as principal components (PCs) which describe most of the information contained in the independent variables in order of decreasing variance. Consequently, PCA reduces dimensionality of a multivariate data set of descriptors to the actual amount of data available. When principal components are employed as the independent variables to perform a linear regression, the method is termed as the principal components regression (PCR). In other words, PCR applies the scores from PCA decomposition as regressors in the QSAR model, to generate a multiple-term linear equation.

Genetic function approximation (GFA) serves as an alternative to standard regression analysis for building QSAR equations. It employs the natural principles of evolution of species which leads to improvements by recombination (mutation and crossover) of independent variables. This method results in multiple models generated by evolving random initial models using genetic algorithm. The method is suitable for obtaining QSAR equations when dealing with a larger number of independent variables. It can build linear as well as higher-order nonlinear equations, perform automatic outlier removal and classification by utilizing spline-based terms.

Genetic partial least squares (G/PLS or GA-PLS) is a valuable analytical tool that has evolved by combining the best features of GFA and PLS, and has been widely preferred by the researchers. In recent years, other methods to perform qualitative or classification studies have been spurred in the field of QSAR. The so-called pattern recognition methods based on the principle of analogy are used for the detection of the distance or closeness within the large amount of multivariate data. It searches for structural features such as the presence (or absence) of certain groups, number of a certain type of atom, or mass spectral-fragmentation so that new compounds can be classified as similar or dissimilar to the members of the existing classes.

Cluster analysis is a statistical pattern recognition method used to investigate the relationship between observations associated with several properties and to partition the data set into categories consisting of similar elements. It allows for the consideration of the inactive compounds in the analysis and can be used to study a large set of substituents to identify which of the subsets share similar physical properties.

The technique of **artificial neural networks (ANNs)** has its origin from the real neurons present in an animal brain. ANNs are parallel computational systems consisting of groups of highly interconnected processing elements called neurons, which are arranged in a series of layers. The first layer is termed the input layer, and each of its neurons receives data from outside/user, corresponding to one of the independent variables used as inputs in QSAR. Subsequent to the input layer, there are one or many layers of neurons, collectively termed as the hidden layers. The last layer is the output layer, and its neurons handle the output from the network. Each layer may make its independent computations and may pass the results yet to another layer. The working of ANNs is given below:

- Each input descriptor value is multiplied by the connection weight, as per its significance
- The weighted inputs are summed up and supplied to the hidden layers, where a nonlinear transfer function does all the required processing
- The results of the transfer function are communicated to the neurons in the output layer, where the results are interpreted and finally presented to the user.

The k-nearest neighbour (kNN) method is one of the simplest machine learning algorithms, most commonly used for classifying a new pattern (e.g. a molecule). The technique is based on a simple distance learning approach whereby an unknown/new molecule is classified according to the majority of its k-nearest neighbours in the training set. The nearness is determined by a Euclidean distance metric (e.g. a similarity measure computed using the structural descriptors of the molecules). Typically, the kNN approach is executed as follows:

- Euclidean distances between an unknown object (u) and all the objects in the training set are computed.
- Based on the calculated distances, k objects from the training set most similar to object u are selected.
- Object u is assigned to the group to which the majority of the k objects belong
- An optimal k value is selected by optimization through the categorization of a test set of samples or by leave-one out cross-validation.

6 | Molecular Modeling— Tool for Drug Design and Molecular Docking

MOLECULAR MODELING

Now-a-days molecular modeling is an important and essential tool to the chemists in the drug design process. Molecular modeling describes the generation, manipulation or demonstration of three-dimensional structures of molecules and associated physicochemical properties. It involves a series of computerized techniques based upon theoretical and experimental data to predict molecular and biological properties. Depending upon the situation and the rigidity, the subject is referred to as 'molecular visualizations', 'molecular graphics', 'computational chemistry', or 'computational quantum chemistry'. The molecular modeling techniques are derived from the concepts of molecular orbitals and classical mechanical programs.

Why Molecular Modeling?

Molecular modeling helps to understand chemistry in a better way by providing advanced techniques for investigating, interpreting, explaining and discovering new phenomena. Molecular modeling helps in the generation, manipulation or representation of three dimensional structures of molecule and associated physiological properties as well. Like experimental chemistry, it is a skill-demanding science and must be learnt by doing and not just reading. Molecular modeling is uncomplicated to execute with currently available software, but the trouble lies in getting the correct model and appropriate interpretation.

Molecular Modeling Tools

The following tools are required for modeling of a drug using computers.

    i. Hardware: A range of classes of computers are necessary for molecular modeling. For chemical information systems the preference of a computer is generally larger, and many packages run on VAX, IBM, or PRIME machines. At present, the molecular modelling chemists are using equipment from manufacturers such as Digital, IBM, Sun, Hewlett-Packard and Silicon Graphics running with the UNIX operating system.

    ii. Software components: A range of commercial packages are available for PC-based systems as well as supercomputer based systems. The computational programmes allow scientists to generate and present molecular data including geometries (bond lengths, bond angles, torsion angles), energies (heat of formation, activation energy, *etc.*) and physical properties (volumes, surface areas, diffusion, viscosity, *etc.*).

Molecular Modeling Methods

At present, two major modeling methods are used for the designing of new drugs. They are:

i. *Direct drug design:* In the direct approach, the three-dimensional features of the known receptor binding site are determined by using X-ray crystallography to design a new lead molecule. In this method, the receptor site geometry is known; the difficulty is to find a molecule that has some geometric constraints and is also a good chemical match. After finding good candidates based upon these criteria, a molecular docking technique with energy minimization can be used to predict binding strength.

ii *Indirect drug design:* The indirect drug design method involves comparative analysis of structural features of known active and inactive molecules that are complementary with a hypothetical receptor site.

Molecular Modeling Applications

Various applications of computer based molecular modeling techniques are as follows:

1. *Generation of chemical structures:* Molecular structures may be created by various softwares. The 3D structures of molecules may be generated by numerous common building functions like make-bond, break-bond, fuse rings, delete-atom, add-atom-hydrogens, put-chiral center, *etc.* Molecular modeling allows chemists to design dynamic models of molecules which consecutively let them to visualize molecular geometry and exhibit chemical principles.

2. *Molecular structure visualization:* The most important area of the molecular modeling concept is visualization of molecular structures and interactions. The molecules are visualized in three dimensions by various illustrations like connected sticks, ball and stick models, space filling representations and surface displays.

3. *Generation of conformations:* The most active area of theoretical research using molecular orbital theory has been in the prediction of the most preferred conformation of molecules. The majority molecules exist in multiple conformations. The preferred conformation of a molecule is a structural characteristic feature that comes up as a response to the force of attraction and repulsion. The shape should be considered primarily in determining the interaction of the molecule with the receptor. The energy minimization is a function of bond angles, bond lengths, torsion angles and non-covalent interactions. By changing these parameters in a systematic way and calculating the total energy as a sum of orbital energies, one can find out a minimum energy structure for example, by using conjugated gradient algorithm working under universal force field.

4. *Modeling of drug receptor interactions:* The 3D structures of many ligands (drug molecules) that interact with the receptors may be known but the structures of most receptors are unknown. The interaction of macromolecular receptors and of small drug molecules is an crucial step in many biological processes such as regulatory mechanisms, pharmacological actions of drugs, the toxic effect of certain chemicals, *etc.* The receptor cavity mode is constructed by using

programmes like RECEPS and AUTO FIT. The receptor model provides 3D information on the physical and chemical properties of the receptor cavity, size, shape of the cavity, H-bond probability and electrostatic potential.

5. *Docking (molecular interactions):* Modeling the binding of a drug with its receptor is a difficult problem. Several forces are involved in the intermolecular association: hydrophobic, van der Waals, dispersion, hydrogen bonding, and electrostatic. The major force for binding appears to be hydrophobic interactions, but the specificity of the binding appears to be controlled by hydrogen bonding and electrostatic interactions. The process of docking a ligand to a binding site tries to mimic the natural course of interaction of the ligand and its receptor via a lowest energy pathway.

6. *Determination of molecular properties:* Molecular properties of chemical molecules including pharmaceuticals are important in various processes. They are normally categorized as physical, chemical and biological. The three major computational methods used for calculation of properties of molecules are:

   i. Empirical (molecular) mechanics: Molecular mechanics methods are less complicated, fast, and are able to handle very large systems including enzymes. Molecular mechanics is a formalism which attempts to reproduce molecular geometries, energies and other features by adjusting bond lengths, bond angles and torsion angles to equilibrium values that are dependent on the hybridization of an atom and its bonding scheme. A force field is used to calculate the energy and geometry of a molecule. It is a collection of atom types, parameters and equations.

   ii. Molecular dynamics: Molecular dynamics simulations are used in various bimolecular applications. This technique, when united with data derived from NMR studies, has been used to derive 3D structures for peptides and small proteins in cases where X-ray crystallography was not practical.

   iii. Quantum mechanics: Quantum mechanics is one of the oldest mathematical expression of theoretical chemistry. In its purest form, quantum theory uses well-known physical constants such as velocity of light, values for the masses and charges of nuclear particles and differential equations to directly calculate molecular properties and geometrics.

7. *Determination of drug excipient interactions:* Molecular modeling technique is used to study the drug-excipient interaction which helps to visualize the type and site of interaction on a computer monitor. It was reported in a study that seven glucose units were combined to get a well shaped energy minimized conformation. The cavity depth, diameter of a wider and narrower rim were calculated and compared to the literature values using DTMM package. Similarly, norfloxacin, ciprofloxacin, *etc.* structures were built to get energy minimized conformation. The dimensions of these molecules were measured and compared to literature values. The drug molecules were allowed to penetrate through the cavity and the probability of penetration was observed. Finally, the success in the formation of inclusion complex of beta cyclodextrin with norfloxacin, ciprofloxacin, tinidazole and methotrexate was reported.

8. *Quantitative structure activity relationship studies:* Quantitative structure activity relationship (QSAR) is a technique that quantifies the relationship between structural and biological properties. A QSAR can be expressed in its most general form by the following equation: Biological activity = f (physicochemical and/or

structural parameters). The physicochemical descriptors include parameters that account for hydrophobicity, topology, electronic properties and steric effects, and are determined empirically by computational methods.

9. *Lead generation:* A lead is any chemical entity which has some biological activity. It is not the same as a drug molecule, but its generation is an important step in drug discovery process. It is the process of identifying potential drug compounds or leads that interact with a target with sufficient potency and selectivity. Lead generation is a difficult process, which involves two basic steps: i) Lead finding: Here the task is to find a chemical entity, which has a desired biological activity. ii) Lead optimization: Lead optimization involves elaborating around the basic lead structure to build in all the desirable properties, such as safety, solubility, efficacy, *etc.*

10. *Determination of properties of pharmacophoric pattern:* A pharmacophoric pattern may be defined as geometrically arranged functionality possessed by a set of active compounds having some mechanism of action. Identification of pharmacophore is specially useful for designing receptor agonists and antagonists, enzyme inhibitors, *etc.* Molecular modeling approach has been already rewarded for the study of dopamine agonists, antagonists and for drugs acting on histamine and morphine receptors.

Molecular Docking

In the drug discovery, high-throughput screening requires the screening of millions of compounds for a particular protein target. The biological research has become increasingly data sensitive. The biomedical projects require latest informatics tools. Molecular docking and database mining are the important tools for improving such screenings. The structure of receptor ligand complexes is predicted by molecular docking. The receptor is generally a protein or a protein oligomer and the ligand is a small molecule or a protein. Initially, molecular docking was used to predict protein-ligand complex structures. To increase the application of molecular docking in different fields many simplifications were done.

Formally, the restrictions in protein-ligand docking came when the description (geometrical and chemical) of the protein and the small organic molecule was not known. Therefore, computational technique is required to check the binding of small molecule to the protein. If it occurs, then we need to know the geometry and the binding affinity of the complex. Mostly algorithms have two components, first, a search technique to find out the best possible position of the ligand in the binding pocket of the protein and second, a scoring function to rate each position, as well as to rank candidate ligands adjacent to each other. Alternatively, we can say that the docking is the process to predict of conformation and orientation (or posing) of a ligand within a targeted binding site. Structural modeling and prediction of activity are two aims of docking studies. But, the prediction of modifications in compound that improve effectiveness and identification of molecular features which are responsible for specific biological identification, are much more complex issues that are usually difficult to understand and simulate on the computer.

Manual Docking

The *dock* or fit a molecule in the binding site. In this, both binding group on the ligand and binding site are known. Ideal bonding distance for potential interaction is defined.

The binding group in the ligand is paired with its complementary group in the binding site. The paired groups are not directly overlaid; they are fitted within preferred bonding distance. Both ligand and protein will remain in same conformation throughout the process. The energy minimization will also remain same. So this is a rigid fit, once a molecule successfully docked fit, optimization is carried out. Different conformations of molecule can be docked in the same way to get the best fit.

Basic Requirement for Docking: 3D Atomistic Representation of the Receptor

To perform molecular docking, we require to have data bank for the search of target with proper PDB (protein data bank) format and a approach to prepare ligand as a PDB file. There are various software's (Discovery studio, *etc.*) available from where the ligand can be made in PDB format. A receptor structure of interest at hand is the precondition so as to perform a structure-based screening task. Most commonly, experimental techniques such as X-ray crystallography or NMR is used for determination of structure of the receptor. For obtaining protein structures the protein structure prediction techniques are used such as homology modeling and 'threading'. When the three dimensional structure of the proteins achieved experimentally or by prediction, it may be analyzed by using various computational techniques. If the function of the protein is unknown, then its structure finding is required for recognized binding sites. Usually the binding site or the function of the protein is identified through reference (e.g. the protein can be chosen from a protein family with known function), or by the crystal of ligand-protein complex. The analysis of the binding-site characteristics and the interactions of the protein with a given ligand provide chances to design the novel ligands (Fig. 6.1).

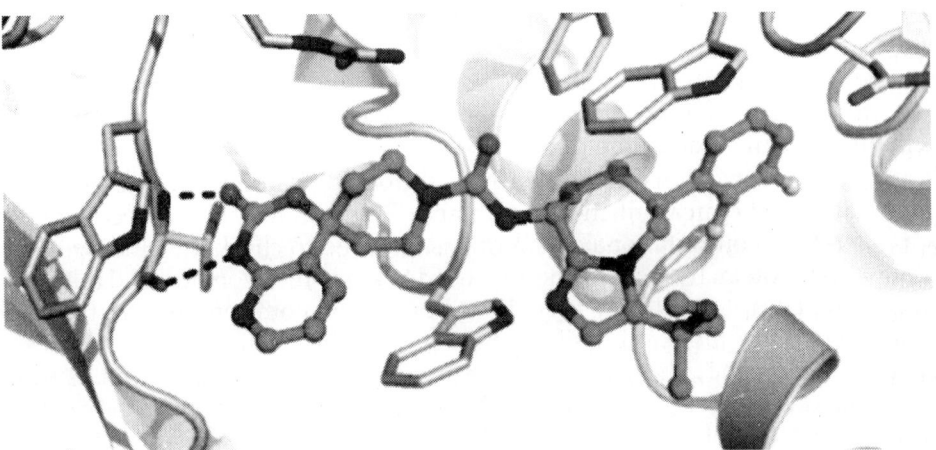

Fig. 6.1: 3D-interaction between ligand and receptor

Docking Scenarios

Docking scenarios typically fall into one of the following categories:
1. When the active site of the protein is unknown, the searching of the binding site as well as the binding mode of the ligand is defined as *blind docking*. It is used for identifying the protein interactions also.

2. When the site of the binding is known from X-ray diffraction or from NMR studies, the docking into the active site is called *direct docking*. In such cases it is possible that:
   - The active site is overlapping with the binding site of a cofactor.
   - The active site contains discrete crystal molecules of water, mediating the binding between the ligand and the target.
   - The active site contains catalytic metal ions.

3. Recent virtual screening techniques deal with some factors such as tautomeric or ionized states of the compounds as well as the effect of the temperature, pK_a, pH, or micro-environment of the active site on ligand binding which are missing in most of the docking approaches.

4. Reproducing the conformational space accessible to a macromolecule is a very difficult task and always necessitates an approximation level:
   - **Rigid body docking:** Both ligand and protein are considered as rigid bodies. Docking procedures that perform rigid body search are termed *rigid docking*.
   - **Semi-flexible docking:** The ligand only is considered flexible.
   - **Fully-flexible docking:** Both ligand and protein are treated as flexible molecules. Docking procedures that consider possible conformational changes are termed **flexible docking**.

Docking is usually a process which has multiple steps and in each step begins one or more supplementary degrees of complexity. Docking search algorithms are the initial step of the process which place (POSE) small molecules in the active site. 'POSING' is defined as the process to determine the specified conformation and orientation of a ligand that placed the active site of the protein. It is generally an indistinct procedure which returns numerous alternative results. Scoring functions are involved with various docking algorithms which are designed to predict the biological activity by evaluating the interactions molecules with the possible targets. Initially scoring functions evaluate the compound interactions with target on the basis of calculations of predicted shape and electrostatic complementarities. Scoring plays its role in both the posing and ranking. The pose score is basically a rough idea to measure of the binding or fixing of a ligand into the active target site. The binding energies may be calculated by rank score, but it is more complex. Ranking is the process that typically takes numerous results from the starting scoring phase and recalculates them. It is more advanced than pose scoring process. This process is generally used to calculate the free energy of binding as precisely as possible. The posing phase uses simple energy calculations (van der Waals and electrostatic) but the ranking methods involves more detailed calculations (properties such as explicit solvation or entropy). Docking procedures are composed of two main components of which the first is a search algorithm and the later is scoring (Fig. 6.2).

1. SEARCH ALGORITHMS

Searching for the Right Pose

Searching for the accurate binding pose of a molecule can be achieved by attempting the number of trials and the poses which are logical in terms of energy, keep those poses for the further process. The search process ends when a number of trials have been attempted and/or an adequate number of poses achieved for a molecule. Docking

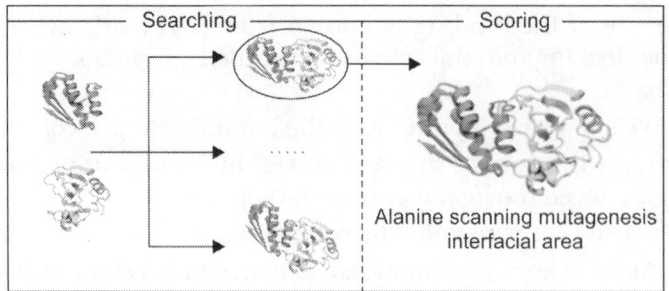

Fig. 6.2: The main docking components—searching and scoring

algorithms have been developed, as discussed in following sections, to maintain the track for previously discovered minima and to find out the new regions.

The accurate binding mode can be discovered by the finding the exact conformation of the docked molecule and the exact orientation because most of the ligand molecules are flexible. Therefore ligand flexibility needs to be handled very carefully. The docking algorithms can be categorized into three types of searches: (a) Systematic (b) Stochastic and (c) Deterministic approaches. Some search algorithms uses combination of these approaches.

a. Systematic Algorithms

In systemic search method, conformations of a molecule are generated by systematically assigned values to the torsion angles of the rotatable bonds. A predetermined set of possible values is produced by each torsion angle. The grid search is the simplest form of systematic search algorithm. It is based on a grid of values for each formal degree of freedom. During the search each of these grid values are explored in a combinatorial manner and conformations related to all promising combinations of torsion angle values are generated. For example, suppose a molecule has two different torsion angles, the first torsion angle has the values 60°, 180° and −60° and the second torsion angle has the values 0° and 180°. The grid search will generate six conformations (i.e. 60,0; 60,180; 180,0; 180,180; −60,0; −60,180). These conformations then one by one subjected to energy minimization. A mathematical equation expresses the grid search, if the number of values permissible to torsion angle is η, and the molecule has N variable torsion angles then the total number of conformations C generated by the grid search would be:

$$C = \Pi_{i=1}^{N} \eta_i$$

So, in a molecule a number of structures will grow exponentially with the number of rotatable bonds. This whole process is sometimes known as a **Combinatorial Explosion**. The algorithms face the problem of combinatorial explosion while they try to search all the degrees of freedom in a molecule. When the number of degrees of freedom increases, simultaneously, the number of evaluations required is also increases. To overcome this situation, a termination criteria is incorporated to avoid the algorithm to get involved in sampling space that leads to the wrong solution.

Thus with the aim to prevent combinatorial explosion in some of these algorithms, the ligand is developed incrementally in the active site, starting from a docked 'base fragment'. A systematic stepwise search can be performed by two different ways:

firstly, by docking the active-site region with different kind of molecular fragments and connecting them covalently (it is referred as the most popular *de novo* ligand-design strategy), secondly, by differentiating docked ligands into core fragment (rigid) and side chains (flexible). In the second case, the identified core fragments which are docked into the active site and the flexible side chains are added in an incremental manner. Representatives of this approach are Hammerhead, DOCK and Flex X. In other approaches, such as Auto Dock, Gold, ICM-Dock and QXP, the ligand is treated in its entirety.

b. Stochastic or Random Search

The random search algorithms are often called stochastic methods which include some kind of repetitious procedure. In this procedure, the structure is selected on the basis of previously generated and randomly modified search and then it is minimized. If this generates a new logical conformation then it is considered in the list of structures found and the process is repeated again. In contrast to the systematic search methods, there is no natural endpoint for a random search or we can say that there is an uncertainty of convergence, this process will continues until either a pre-defined number of trials have been carried out and/or until there is no new conformations can be produced. In other words we can say that in order to improve convergence, multiple, independent runs should be performed. Various random search procedures can be differentiated in two ways: by the structural modification method and by the method of selection of the structure for the next repetition. Modifications can be achieved most commonly either by changing the torsion angles (keeping the bond angles and lengths fixed) or by changing the (xyz) coordinates of the atoms. The simplest method to select the structure for the next repetition is to use the structure generated in the earlier step, however, other methods are also available. An alternative way is to choose the structures randomly which are generated already. This was all about the random search algorithm and it provides three most popular random approaches which are (i) Monte Carlo (ii) Genetic algorithms and (iii) Tabu search algorithms.

i. **The metropolis Monte Carlo scheme:** The Monte Carlo scheme can also be used for the selection. In this, when the new structure has the lower energy (V_{new}) than its predecessor enery (V_{old}) then it can be used as the next starting structure. The Boltzmann factor, $\exp[(V_{new}-V_{old})/kT]$, is calculated ($k$ is the Boltzmann constant and T is the temperature), when V_{new} is higher than the V_{old}. The new structure is selected, if the Boltzmann factor is larger than a random number between zero and one and if it is not, then the previous structure is taken. Thus the Monte Carlo Metropolis method makes it possible that the structures having higher energies can be selected and these can be correlated to the previously unknown areas of conformational space.

Simulated annealing is the most commonly used version of *Monte Carlo* method. In this method, the temperature decreases steadily from a high value to the lower value. The system can overcome the high energy barriers at the high temperatures due to the presence of temperatures in the denominator of the Boltzman factor and this result to discover the search space widely. When the temperature decreases, the lower energy states become viable. At absolute zero temperature, the computational system should exist in the global minimum-energy state by using the physical process of annealing in the manufacture of very large single crystals of materials, for instance, silicon. The global minimum energy conformation is related to the conformational analysis, though, it requires an infinite number of temperature decreases and for each of them the system has to come in equilibrium. Therefore practically it is not mandatory that a system will find the global energy minimum. Thus several simulated annealing runs have to be performed. Alternative implementations of Monte Carlo search have been reported earlier including a popular type in auto dock.

ii. **Genetic algorithms:** Genetic algorithms are the set of computational problem-solving approaches which involves the principles of population dynamics and biological struggle. 'Chromosome' encoded the model parameters which are differentiated stochastically. Chromosomes provide the feasible solutions to a given problem which can be analysed through the fitness function. The chromosomes, responsible for the best intermediate solutions, subjected to crossover dry mutation operations (similar to gene recombination and mutation) to produce the next generation. The genetic algorithm solution is a collection of possible ligand conformations for docking applications. Several programs for example DOCK and GOLD have implemented genetic algorithms.

iii. **Tabu search algorithm:** The tabu search algorithm technique is applicable for the already explored areas of conformational space. The root mean square deviation is calculated between current molecular coordinates and every molecule's previously recorded conformation. It is required to know that a molecular conformation is accepted or not, PRO_LEADS is an example for making the use of a tabu search algorithm.

Tabu search algorithm usually :
- Make little random changes to the existing conformation.
- Rank each change according to the value of the selected fitness function.
- Determine which changes are 'tabu' (that is, earlier rejected conformations).
- If any modification gives the lower value than any other accepted modification then accept it, even if it is in 'tabu'. Or else accept the best 'non-tabu' modification.
- Add the accepted modification to the 'tabu' list and record its score.
- Go to the first step.

c. Deterministic Search/Simulation Methods

In deterministic searches, the initial state determines the progress that can be made to produce the next state. This state should have equal to or lower in energy than the initial state. Deterministic searches performed precisely on the same starting system, including each degree of freedom, with the same parameters which produce exactly the same final state. A problem which usually comes in deterministic algorithms is that they frequently get trapped in local minima because they cannot cross the barriers. To increase capability, for crossing the barriers or to decrease the height of the energy barriers various approaches were tried. Instances of deterministic methods are molecular dynamics (MD) simulations and energy minimization methods.

Molecular dynamics simulation—It is concerned with the atoms of the system and solves the Newton's equations of motion. It is related to the positions of the atoms, how they changes with times. Pictures taken from the sequence may be considered in the minimization, in order to make a sequence of minimum energy conformations. The MD docking algorithm is the combination of changes in temperatures and the degrees of freedom of the system. The two temperatures which are responsible for calculating the flexibility of the ligand can be vary at the time of simulation process. It helps the system to avoid the trapping in a local minimum.

d. Energy Minimization Method

Discussed in Chapter – 11.

2. SCORING

Ligand scoring method is applicable for calculating the binding affinity of a ligand. The binding affinity of candidate ligand is evaluated when it is docked in the binding site of the target receptor structure. The computed ligand–receptor interaction energy (score) of a pose takes the decision for trial pose. 'Dock score' is calculated by many programs to recognize and giving rank order to various poses of a molecule during the search. It is a score based on a simple energy function such as a force field with an electrostatic term, repulsive and attractive van der Waals terms. This can be calculated very easily during the docking process, whereas, more sophisticated function is used to calculate the final 'affinity score' for that molecule.

Scoring Methods and Scoring Functions

Wide ranges of scoring function systems are available now-a-day. They mostly divided into two main categories (Fig. 6.3). The first category includes scoring schemes based on force field physical interaction terms (i.e. van der Waals interactions or hydrogen bonding). This category is further divided in two groups: (a) the 'empirical' scoring functions in which each of the terms are multiplied with a coefficient, the resultant products are summed up to provide the final score. The coefficients are optimized to provide a good fit to the training set of molecules. (b) the 'first- principle-based' scoring functions, in this, the terms are directly derived from physicochemical theory which are not included in experimental data.

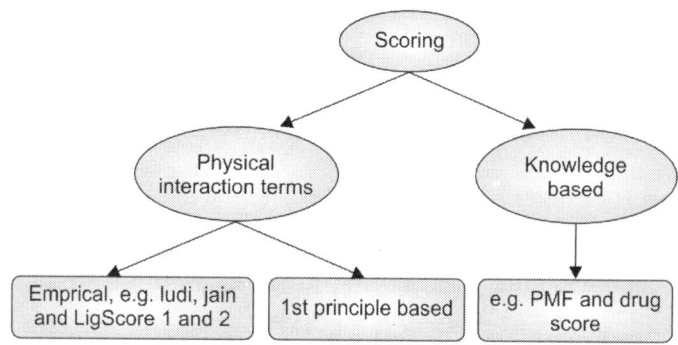

Fig. 6.3: Different types of scoring function schemes

The second category includes 'knowledge-based' scoring functions. These functions can be obtained by applying statistics in the frequencies of the observed inter–atomic contact and distances in crystal structures of protein–ligand complexes. The scoring functions which fall into this category are such as PMF and Drug Score. Many scoring functions can be combined to make a single scoring scheme, this method simplifies the process and this is known as 'consensus score'. In this particular case, a molecule has to score well across the many different scoring schemes to find out an active target binder. Scoring methods typically use empirical functions, as discussed before, which are developed by fitting various functional forms and characterize various aspects of the ligand-receptor interactions against binding affinity data. However, for statistical analysis of known ligand–receptor structures, knowledge based approach is used. It is also used to estimate the frequency of occurrence of specific receptor–ligand interactions without the help of binding affinity information.

The types of scoring functions (from both categories) are as follows:

- Jain
- LigScore 1
- LigScore 2
- Ludi
- Piecewase Linear Potential (PLP)
- Potential of Mean Force (PMF)

The first four scoring functions come under the empirical based approach and the PMF function come under the knowledge-based statistical approach. The scoring function which is correlated well with binding affinities is PLP. It was originally developed as a docking function.

Jain Scoring Function

AN Jain developed an empirical scoring function for the evaluation of the structures as well as binding affinities of protein–ligand complexes. The Jain score is a sum of five interaction terms. These terms describe:

1. Lipophilic interactions
2. Polar repulsive interactions
3. Polar attractive interactions
4. An entropy term for the ligand
5. Solvation of the ligand and protein

For the pairwise interactions, only proximate ligand-protein atoms are considered. The sum of a Gaussian and a sigmoidal function represents the lipophilic and polar interactions. This functional form is short-ranged with a pronounced maximum that occurs at close surface contacts and this also incurs a significant penalty for short contacts between ligand and protein atoms. Options are provided to ignore non-polar hydrogens of the receptor or ignore water molecules when calculating the Jain score.

LigScore Scoring Function

Lig Score scoring functions are further of two types Lig Score 1 and Lig Score 2.

a. **LigScore 1** is the simple, fast, scoring function used for predicting the binding affinity of ligand-receptor complex. Three descriptors are involved to calculate Lig Score1 and expressed in units of pK_i ($-\log K_i$). These descriptors are:

- vdW: It is a softened Lennard–Jones 6-9 potential. It is expressed in units of kcal/mol.
- C+pol: It calculates the buried polar surface area between a ligand and receptor which holds attractive ligand-receptor interactions. It expressed in units of $Å^2$.
- TotPol^2: It is the squared sum of the total polar surface area of the ligand and receptor and expressed in units of $Å^2$.

The individual inputs of these descriptors are also available along with the overall LigScore 1 value during the scoring. LigScore1 calculated by using two different kinds of equation depending upon the forcefield (CFF or DREIDING) employed for the calculation of the vdW descriptor which corresponds to the charge model (Gastieger or CFF) used to assign atoms as polar or nonpolar. The corresponding LigScorel equations are:

$$\text{LigScorel\_CFF} = 0.4896 - 0.04551*vdW + 0.1439*C+pol - 0.00.1010*TotPol^2 \tag{6.1}$$

$$\text{LigScorel\_Dreiding} = -0.3498 - 0.04673*vdW + 0.1653*C+pol - 0.001132*TotPol^2 \tag{6.2}$$

where, the coefficients were achieved by regression analysis of the binding affinities of a series of ligand-protein-complexes.

   b. **LigScore 2** is also the simple and fast scoring function for predicting the binding affinity of ligand-receptor complex. In this also, three descriptors are involved to calculate LigScore 2 and expressed in the units of pk_i ($-\log K_i$). These descriptors are:

   • vdW: It is a softened Lennard–Jones 6-9 potential. It is expressed in units of kcal/mol.
   • C+pol: It calculates the buried polar surface area between a ligand and receptor which holds attractive ligand-receptor interactions. It expressed in units of $Å^2$.
   • Bury Pol^2: It is the squared sum of the buried polar surface area of the ligand and receptor and expressed in units of $Å^2$. It is used for the desolvation penalty invited by desolvating water molecules from the receptor and ligand binding space so that the ligand can bind to the receptor.

The individual inputs of these descriptors are also available along with the overall LigScore 2 value during the scoring. Like LigScore1, LigScore 2 is calculated by using two different kinds of equation depending upon the forcefield (CFF or DREIDING) employed for the calculation of the vdW descriptor. The current LigScore2 equations are:

$$\text{LigScore2\_CFF} = 1.900 - 0.0730*vdW + 0.06246*C+pol - 0.00007324*BuryPol^2 \tag{6.3}$$

$$\text{LigScore2\_Dreiding} = 1.539 - 0.07622*vdW + 0.6501*C+pol - 0.00007821 *BuryPol^2 \tag{6.4}$$

Where, the coefficients were achieved by regression analysis of the binding affinities of a series of ligand-protein-complexes.

Ludi Scoring Function

The empirical scoring functions provided for the Ludi algorithm are used to evaluate the receptor-ligand interactions. The Ludi score is the sum of five contributions:
   • Ideal hydrogen bonds contribution.
   • The ionic interaction contribution (It is the interaction of donor/acceptor in the receptor [e.g. COO, or $-NH_3^-$]).
   • Lipophilic interactions contribution
   • The freezing of internal degrees of freedom of the ligand contribution.
   • The loss of translational and rotational entropy of the ligand contribution

This scoring function known as *Energy_Estimate_1* derived from the empirically fitting a set of ligand-protein complexes with the binding affinities, which are experimentally achieved. A second scoring function known as *Energy_Estimate_2* calculated by using additional complexes and refitting the weights related previously described terms. A final scoring function known as *Energy_Estimate_3* derived from the same set of complexes used for *Energy_Estimate_2* and including the additional contribution of the aromatic-aromatic interactions in the function.

Piecewise Linear Potential (PLP)

Piecewise Linear Potential is also a simple and fast docking function which evaluates the binding affinities of ligand-protein complexes. PLP scores are measured in arbitrary units. The negative PLP scores are used in the calculations of consensus score. The higher PLP values represent the stronger ligand-receptor binding (larger pK_i values). Two types of the PLP function are available: PLP1 and PLP2.

(a) **PLP1:** In this scoring function, the every non-hydrogen receptor or non-hydrogen ligand atom is considered as a PLP atom. Hydrogens are excluded at the time of scoring. There are four types of PLP atoms:

1. H-bond acceptor only
2. Hydrogen bond (H-bond) donor only.
3. Both H-bond donor and acceptor.
4. Non-polar.

Note: When PLP1 is used, for every new ligand conformation the internal energy will be calculated. This energy is used only to prevent the vander Waals clashes and is not used for the PLP scoring. The forcefield used in this for providing the atomic parameters is generally the robust DREIDING.

The PLP1 score is the sum of the function values of all pairwise interactions in a ligand-receptor complex. H-bond and steric interaction are two types of pairwise interactions included in PLP1 as shown in Table 6.1. These interactions can be explained by the same functional form, but with different parameters (Table 6.2).

Table 6.1: Interaction types of PLP1

Ligand PLP type	Receptor PLP type			
	Donor	*Acceptor*	*Both*	*Non polar*
Donor	Steric	H-bond	H-bond	Steric
Acceptor	H-bond	Steric	H-bond	Steric
Both	H-bond	H-bond	H-bond	Steric
Non-polar	Steric	Steric	Steric	Steric

Table 6.2: Parameters for PLP1 functional form

Interaction type	A	B	C	D	E	F
H-bond	2.3	2.6	3.1	3.4	−2.0	20.00
Steric	3.4	3.6	4.5	5.5	−0.4	20.0

(b) **PLP2:** In this function, the PLP atom typing will remain the same as in PLP1, but the atomic radius for hydrogen atom is not considered.

Three types different radii are:
1. Small   : a value of 1.4 for F and metal ions (including Zn, Mn, Mg, and Fe).
2. Medium : a value of 1.8 for C and N.
3. Large   : a value of 2.2 for S, P, Cl, and Br.

The PLP2 score is the sum of the function values of all pairwise interactions in a receptor-ligand complex. The H- bond, dispersion, and repulsion are three types of pairwise interactions present in PLP2 as shown in Table 6.3. The H-bond and dispersion interactions have the different parameters, but same functional form. A scaling factor is used for H-bond and repulsion interactions based on the angle formed by the corresponding ligand-receptor atoms.

Table 6.3 Interaction types of PLP2				
Ligand PLP type	*Receptor PLP type*			
	Donor	*Acceptor*	*Both*	*Non-polar*
Donor	Repulsion	H-bond	H-bond	Dispersion
Acceptor	H-bond	Repulsion	H-bond	Dispersion
Both	H-bond	H-bond	H-bond	Dispersion
Non-polar	Dispersion	Dispersion	Dispersion	Dispersion

1. Pairwise potential for H-bond and dispersion terms.
2. Pairwise potential for repulsion terms.
3. Scaling factor for H-bond and repulsion interactions based on the angle formed by the receptor and ligand atoms.

Potential of Mean Force (PMF)

The PMF and PMF04 scoring functions are designed on the basis of statistical analysis of the 3D structures of ligand-protein complexes. They are simple and fast scoring functions concerned with the protein–ligand binding free energies calculations. The scores are the total sum of pairwise interactions with over all inter-atomic pairs of the ligand-receptor complex. PMF04 score is the upgraded version of the previous PMF score. For the evaluation a large set of data is required and additionally, halogen potentials and metal ions are also involved. The PMF scores are measured in arbitrary units. The negative score value used in the calculation of consensus score. The higher values represent the stronger ligand-receptor binding affinity. To ensure accurate atom typing for the PMF calculation, the correct bond order information is required and the hydrogen atoms are excluded from the ligand and receptor structures. While the hydrogen atom type was included in the parameterization scheme for PMF, it can be ignored during the score calculation. Options are also available for setting distance cutoffs for the calculation of carbon–carbon interactions and other interactions as discussed by Muegge and Martin.

Influence of Forcefield, Partial and Formal Charges on Scoring Functions

Several of the available scoring functions depend on the values of atom charges (both partial and formal) and also the choice of forcefield. Atom partial charges are automatically recalculated when performing a scoring calculation, and these partial charges depend on the forcefield choice. Any previously calculated partial charges are ignored in scoring calculations. Two forcefields are available when calculating ligand-protein scores, CFF and DREIDING. If CFF is chosen, then partial charges will be assigned to all atoms of the ligand and protein based on the CFF charging rules. If DREIDING is selected, then the Gasteiger charging method will be employed to calculate the partial charges of ligands and proteins. The forcefield selected will also affect the vander Waals energy term used in both LigScore1 and LigScore2.

- LigScore1 uses the partial charges on the atoms of both ligand and receptor to determine whether an atom is polar or nonpolar based on a cutoff threshold. This influences the computation of C+Pol and TotPol2.
- LigScore2 types atoms of ligands and proteins as polar or nonpolar based on rules that employ only formal charges, ignoring partial charges.
- PLP1 and PLP2 do not use any charge information, so partial charges, formal charges, and forcefield have no effect on the computed scores.
- The Jain scoring function depends explicitly on the formal charge values in the polar attractive and repulsive interaction terms. The function is independent for both partial charges and forcefield.
- The PMF and Ludi scoring functions depend implicitly on formal charges in their atom typing assignment rules, but are independent of partial charges or forcefield.

The major aim at the end of docking is to reach a druggable site and in order to assess it following are the major parameters which need to be considered as shown in Table 6.4.

Table 6.4: Parameters considered for identifying a druggable site

Parameter	Ideal value	Explanation
Shape	Deep or enclosed	The ligned-receptor interaction energy roughly correlates with the surface contact area.
Size	Fits ligands of 300–600 Da	Small molecules require enveloping cavities to attain sufficient binding affinity. Small cavities may not be able to accommodate drug like molecules. Very large cavities may not provide sufficient surface contact area.
Chemical Character	Mix of hydrophobic and hydrophilic	Drug molecules present a balance between lipophilicity (low log P) and hydrophilicity (H-bond donor/acceptors, PSA).
Flexibility	Rigid	Binding to very flexible binding sites involves an entropic penalty. Flexibility of the receptor is a difficult property to handle.

Besides the difficulties associated with the scoring of compound conformations, there are other complications exist which demands to predict the accurate conformations for binding and biological activity of compound. These are such as limited resolution of crystallographic targets, induced fit, inherent flexibility, other conformational changes which occur on binding, and the participation of water molecules in ligand-protein interactions. The docking is scientifically complex process.

Pose Prediction versus Affinity Prediction

The 'docking' is referred as the placing of the molecules in the receptor-binding site, but the 'scoring' is referred as the prediction of affinity of the binding. Now a day the docking programs are designed to perform both the actions. Technically the two major challenges are faced by docking programs due to the variations in docking and scoring functions: First, the prediction of the molecule's binding mode accurately called as 'pose prediction' (Pose refers to the molecule's conformation and orientation at the receptor target binding site). Second, the binding affinity prediction of the compounds or to generate the comparative rank-ordering for a number of compounds used to target binding site in a consistent manner.

Analysis of Poses

There are number of protocols available in DS2.5 (Discovery Studio 2.5, molecular ducking software) for analyzing the poses, all found under Receptor Ligand Interactions. Some of them are Analyse Ligand Poses where calculation of RMSD of the poses and the analysis of contacts between the ligand and the receptor is done; Calculate Binding Energies; Calculate Interaction Energies, *etc.* All the protocols are run in similar manner by entering the required parameters in the specified protocol as discussed above for docking and scoring protocols.

Applications of Molecular Docking

Molecular docking can specify the feasibility of any biochemical reaction as it is carried out before experimental part of any investigation. There are some areas, where molecular docking has transformed the findings, particularly in the interaction between small molecules (ligand) and protein target (may be an enzyme) may predict the activation or inhibition of enzyme. Such type of information may provide a raw material for the rational drug designing. Some of the major applications of molecular docking are described below:

 i. **Lead optimization:** Molecular docking can predict an *optimized orientation* of ligand on its target. It can predict different binding modes of ligand in the groove of target lead molecule. This can be used to build up more potent, selective and efficient drug molecules.

 ii. **Hit identifications:** Docking with scoring function may be used to *assess large databases* for finding out potent drug molecule *in silico*, which can target the binding site of interest.

iii. **Drug DNA interaction:** Molecular docking plays a important role in the initial prediction of drug's binding properties to nucleic acid. This information establishes the correlation between drug's molecular structure and its cytotoxicity. Keeping this in mind, medicinal chemists are continuously putting their efforts to explain the underlying anticancer mechanism of drugs at molecular level by investigating the interaction mode between nucleic acid and drugs in presence of copper. Medicinal chemists are doing *in silico* observations where their main focus is to find whether the drug is bonding with the protein/DNA. If the docking programme is finding any success in the said interaction, then the experimental procedures are made available to find out the real binding mode of the complex. This leads to the development of new anticancer drug.

Basic Challenges in Molecular Docking

Certain basic challenges in docking and scoring are discussed under the following headings.

i. **Ligand chemistry:** The ligand preparation has important effect on the docking results because the ligand recognition by any biomolecule depends on 3D structure orientation and electrostatic interaction. This shows that the conformation of both the ligand as well as ligand preparation is important. Earlier, keeping estimated pKa values, the structure being most likely optimized by removing or adding hydrogens but the tautomeric and protomeric states of the molecules which are to be docked, still remained a major problem. Since almost all databases keep molecules in their neutral forms but under physiological conditions they are actually ionized. Hence, it is mandatory to ionize them prior to docking. But in different programs, the standard ionization is easy to get. Regarding the issue of tautomers, the problem still remains there, which tautomer one should use or should one use all possible tautomers.

ii. **Receptor flexibility:** This is a foremost challenge in docking, i.e. handling of flexible protein. A protein structure has different conformations depending upon the ligand to which it interacts. This shows that docking performed with a rigid receptor will give a single conformation of receptor. However, when the docking process is performed with flexible receptor, the ligands may require many receptor conformations to interact. In molecular docking studies, usually the most neglected side is *different conformational* states of proteins. Since the protein flexibility is essential as it accounts for better affinity to be achieved between a given drug and target. Another issue of target flexibility is active site water molecules, they must be removed to avoid using artefact waters in the docking process.

iii. **Scoring function:** Another challenge in docking is imperfection in scoring function. Just like search algorithm (able to give optimum conformation), scoring function should also be able to differentiate true binding modes from all the other parallel modes. A potential scoring function would be computationally much economical, unfavourable for analyzing several binding modes. When there is precision, scoring functions make numerous suggestions to calculate ligand affinity. The physical phenomenon, i.e., entropy and electrostatic interactions are disregarded in scoring functions. Hence, the lack of suitable scoring function, both in terms of accuracy and speed, is the main obstruction in molecular docking programming.

DE NOVO DRUG DESIGN

De novo means start a fresh, from the beginning, from the scratch. It is a process in which the 3D structure of receptor is used to design newer molecules. It involves structural determination of the lead target complexes and lead modifications using molecular modeling tools (Fig. 6.4). Information about target receptor is available but not about existing lead compound that can interact with the receptor.

Principles of *De Novo* Drug Design

- Assembling possible compounds and evaluating their quality.
- Searching the sample space for novel structures with drug like properties.
- Build model of binding site protein structure.

Protien structure   Build model of binding site   Construct molecule that fits the model

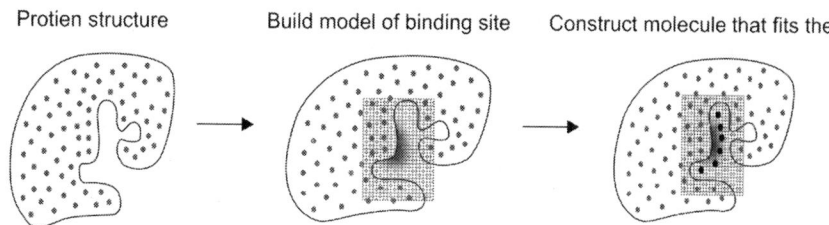

Fig. 6.4: *De novo* drug design

Computer-based Drug Design Consists of the Following Steps

1. Generation of potential primary target constraints
2. Derivation of interaction sites
3. Building up methods
4. Assay (or) scoring
5. Search strategies
6. Secondary target constraints

1. Primary Target Constraints

These are the molecules which set up a framework for the desired structure with the required ligand receptor interactions - These are of 2 types: (i) receptor based: interactions of the receptor form basis for the drug design. (ii) ligand based: ligand to the target functions as a key.

In *de novo* design, the structure of the target should be known to a high resolution, and the binding to site must be well defined. This should defines not only a shape constraint but hypothetical interaction sites, typically consisting of hydrogen bonds, electrostatic and other non-covalent interactions. These can greatly reducing the sample space, as hydrogen bonds and other anisotropic interactions can define specific orientations.

2. Derivation of Interaction Sites

It is a key step to model any binding site as accurately as possible. This starts with an atomic resolution structure of the active site. Programs like UCSF, DOCK define the volume available to a ligand by filling the active site with spheres. Further constraints follow, using positions of H-bond acceptors and donors. Other docking algorithms, such as FLOG, GOLD, and FlexiDock 16 use an all-atom representations to achieve fine detail. Ray-tracing algorithms, such as SMART represent another strategy.

3. Building-up Strategies

a. Growing: A single key building block is the starting point or seed. Fragments are added to provide suitable interactions to both key sites and space between key sites. These include simple hydrocarbon chains, amines, alcohols, and even single rings. In the case of multiple seeds, growth is usually simultaneous and continues until all pieces have been integrated into a single molecule (Fig. 6.5).

b. Linking: The fragments, atoms, or building blocks are either placed at key interaction sites (or) pre-docked using another program. They are joined together using pre-defined rules to yield a complete molecule. Linking groups or linkers may be predefined or generated to satisfy all required conditions (Fig. 6.6).

c. Lattice based method: The lattice is placed in the binding site, and atoms around key interaction sites are joined using the shortest path. Then various iterations, each of which includes translation, rotation or mutation of atoms, are guided by a potential energy function, eventually leading to a target molecule.

d. Molecular dynamics methods: The building blocks are initially randomly placed and then by MD simulations allowed to rearrange. After each rearrangement certain bonds were broken and the process repeated. During this procedure high scoring structures were stored for later evaluation.

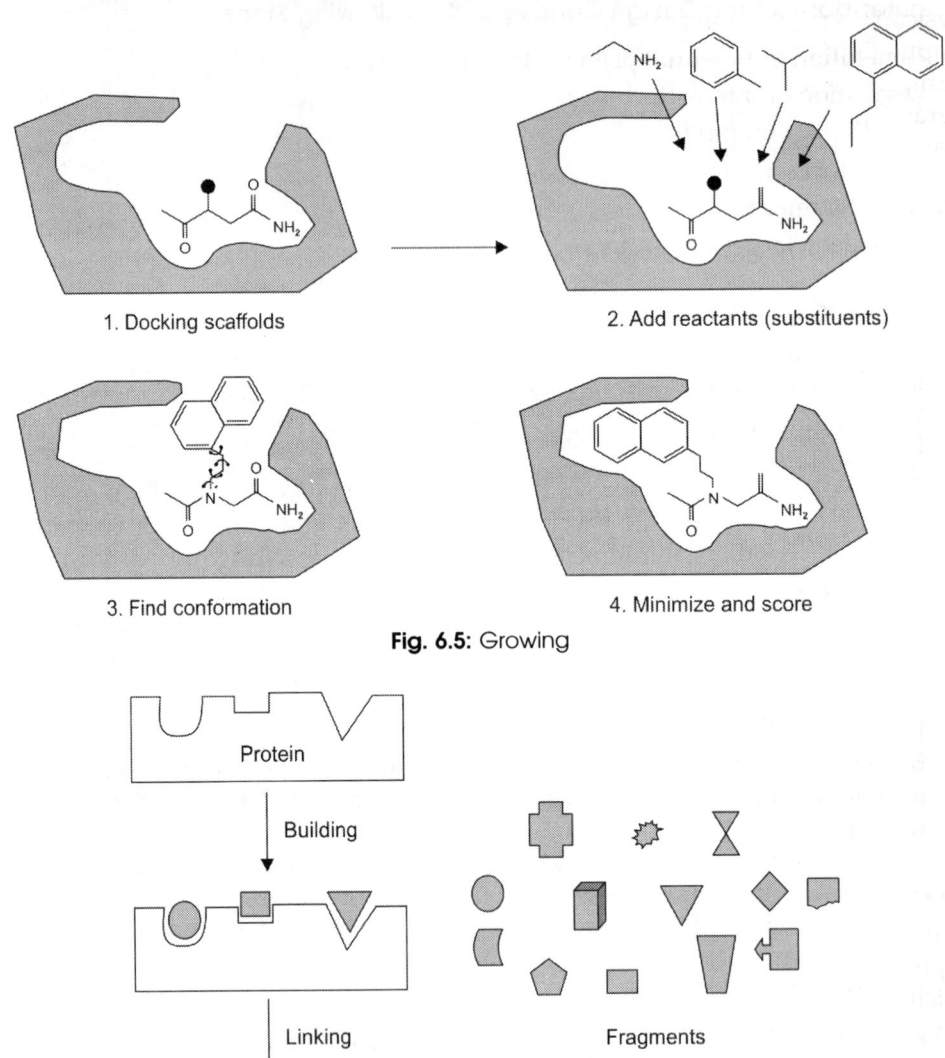

1. Docking scaffolds

2. Add reactants (substituents)

3. Find conformation

4. Minimize and score

Fig. 6.5: Growing

Protein

Building

Linking

Fragments

Fig. 6.6: Linking

4. Scoring

Each solution should be tested to decide which is the most promising, this is called as scoring. Programs such as LEGEND18, LUDI19, Leap-Frog16, SPROUT20, HOOK21, and PRO-LIGAND22 are using different scoring techniques. These scoring functions vary from simple steric constraints and H-bond placement to explicit force fields and empirical or knowledge-based scoring methods. Programs like GRID and LigBuilder3 set up a grid in the binding site and then assess interaction energies by placing probe atoms or fragments at each grid point. Scoring functions guide the growth and optimization of structures by assigning fitness values to the sampled space. Scoring functions attempt to approximate the binding free energy by substituting the exact physical model with simplified statistical methods. Force fields usually involve more computation than the other types of scoring functions, e.g. LEGEND

Empirical scoring functions are a weighted sum of individual ligand–receptor interactions. Apart from scoring functions, attempts have been made to use NMR, X-ray analysis and MS to validate the fragments.

5. Search Strategies

Types of search strategies are as follows:
a. Combinatorial search algorithms: It reduces the effective size of the solution space and explores the space efficiently.
b. Breadth first: It keeps all possible solutions per step, and solves them all to end structures. This can only be done in a limited fashion, as an exhaustive search would not be feasible.
c. Depth first: It selects the highest scoring solution per step and then proceeds. This strategy may spontaneously generate nonsense solutions. Usually combinations of these last two are used; for example, a breadth-first search could be done until the solution space is relatively limited and in subsequent steps depth- first searches would be used.
d. Monte Carlo algorithms: This function based on random sampling, and are usually tied with the "Metropolis criterion". After each modification, the partial solution is either accepted if it is a better solution or rejected, based upon the difference of scoring of the modified versus the unmodified structure.
e. Evolutionary Algorithms: It models natural processes, such as selection, recombination, mutation, and migration, and work in a parallel manner. The number of partial solutions is not fixed and "evolves" based on the "fitness" of the solutions.

6. Secondary Target Constraints

Binding affinity alone does not suffice to make an effective drug molecule. Essential properties include effective Absorption, Distribution, Metabolism, Excretion and Toxicity (ADMET).

In general, an orally active drug has:
a. Not more than 5 hydrogen bond donors (OH and NH groups),
b. Not more than 10 hydrogen bond acceptors (notably N and O),
c. A molecular weight under 500 Da
d. A log P (log ratio of the concentrations of the solute in the solvent) under 5.

Using these rules as a filter, the resulting compounds are more likely to have biological activity.

7 | Virtual Screening Techniques

INTRODUCTION

Drug discovery is all about finding new molecules that interact in a desired way with target, namely proteins and other macromolecules in the human body. If the 3D structures of both small and large molecules are known, they can be tested with a reasonable degree of accuracy. The virtual screening can be applied to all those yet to be synthesized compounds.

Virtual screening is a computer based *technique,* used in drug discovery to search libraries of small molecules in order to identify those structures which are most likely to bind to a drug target, usually a protein receptor or enzyme.

Computational screening of databases has become gradually more fashionable in the pharmaceutical research. Virtual screening uses computer based methods to discover new ligands on the basis of biological structures. Virtual screening is divided into *structural based screening (docking)* as shown in Fig. 7.1 and *screening using active compounds as templates (ligand based virtual screening)*. Ligand based screening techniques principally focus on comparing molecular similarity analysis of compounds with known and unknown moiety, regardless of the methods of the used algorithm. Docking is a computational tool of structure based drug design to predict protein ligand interaction geometries and binding affinities. In this chapter, we will give an overview of the previously used ligand based virtual screening and the docking with a range of databases, filters, scores and applications in the modern research in the pharmaceutical sector.

DRUG LIKENESS SCREENING

Many drug molecules fail in the clinical trials, the reasons behind this are unrelated to the potency against the desired drug target. Pharmacokinetic properties and toxicity issues are blamed for more than half of all failure in the clinical trials. Therefore, first part of the virtual screening evaluates *druglikeness* of small molecules, drug like molecules exhibit favourable absorption, distribution, metabolism, excretion and toxicological (ADMET) parameters. Following types of method currently used to calculate druglikeness:

1. Simple counting method
2. Functional group filter
3. Topological filter
4. Pharmacophore filter

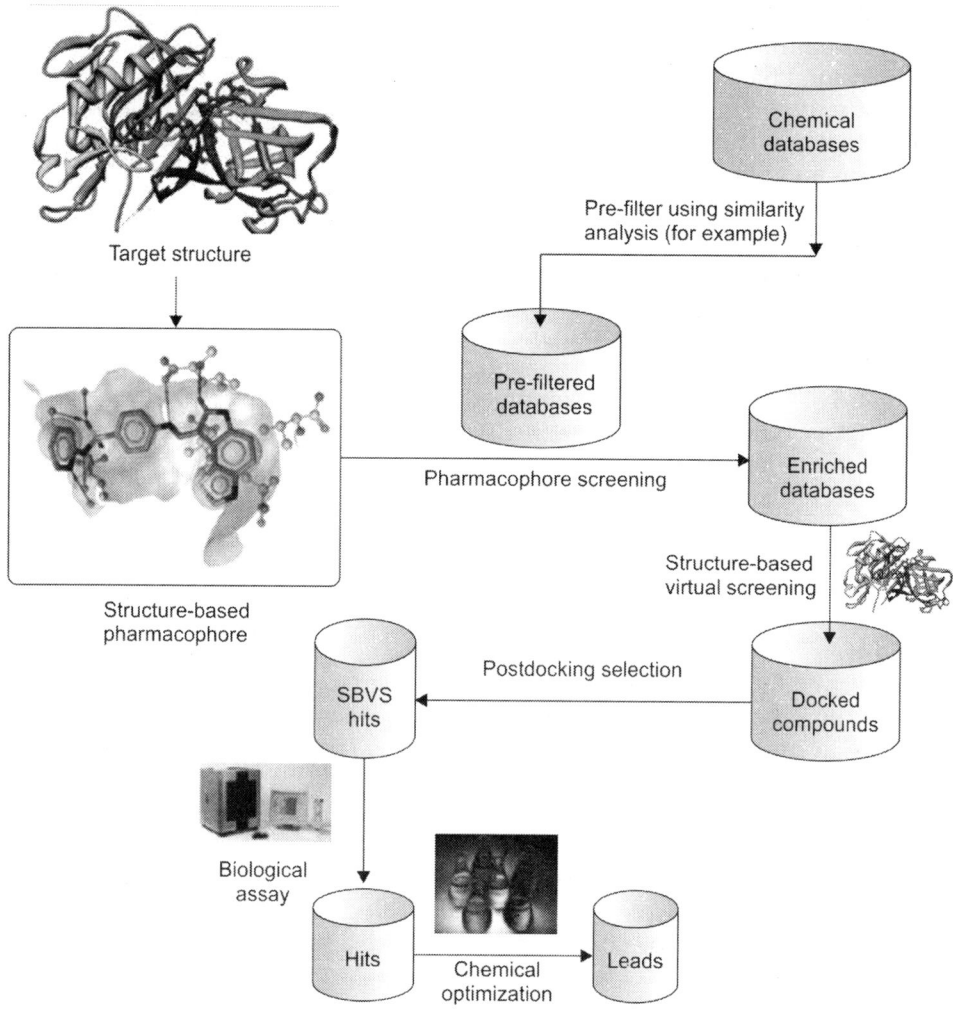

Fig. 7.1: Typical structure-based virtual screening-based drug development protocol

1. **Simple counting method:** Database collections of known drug are generally used to find out structural properties of potential drug molecules. Molecular weight, charge and lipophilicity are contoured to take out simple counting rules for significant description of ADMET- related parameters.

2. **Functional group filter:** Unsuitable, reactive and toxic compounds, such as natural product derivatives, are removed using specific filters. Typical reactive functional groups like alkyl halide peroxide, carbazide, ethers, disulphide, and aliphatic methylene chain having seven or more carbons and unsuitable natural products like quinones, polyenes, and cycloheximidine derivative can be removed by using filters. Screenings out the compound that contain definite atom groups associated with toxicity provide a practical and fast way to diminish large database. Better explanation of toxicity may provide structure-based method to calculate toxicity of the compound.

3. **Topological drug filter:** It is usually assumed that compound those having the structure similarity with known drug may show drug like properties themselves, such as oral bioavailability, low toxicity, membrane permeability and metabolic stability. Its first part, artificial neural networks and decision trees are very fast filter tool in virtual screening approaches. Data's also collected to find structural patterns and pharmacophore features of small molecules that characterize drugs. For the analysis of virtual libraries according to the presence or absence of drug like framework, side chain or structural patterns can be used for virtual screening.

4. **Pharmacophore filter:** It is based on the assumption that drug like molecules should contain at least two distinct pharmacophore groups, four functional designs have been identified that guarantee hydrogen bonding capability which are important for the specific interaction of the drug molecules with its biological target. These designs can be combined to substituent groups that are also called as pharmacophore points; these include: amine, amide, alcohol, ketone, sulphone, sulphonamide, carboxylic acid carbamate, guanidine, amidine, urea, and ester.

Pharmacophore

Historical perspective: The idea of the pharmacophore was developed by Paul Ehrlich during the late 1800s. At that time, the certain "chemical groups" or functions in a molecule were considered responsible for a biological effect, and molecules with similar effect had similar functions in general. The word pharmacophore was given much later, by Schueler in his 1960 book *Chemobiodynamics and Drug Design*, and was defined as "a molecular framework that carries (phoros) the essential features responsible for a drug's (pharmacon) biological activity." The definition of a pharmacophore was therefore no longer concerned with "chemical groups" but "patterns of abstract features." Since 1997, a pharmacophore has been defined by the International Union of Pure and Applied Chemistry as:

A pharmacophore is the collection of steric and electronic features that is required to ensure the optimal supramolecular interactions with a specific biological target and to trigger (or block) its biological response.

Pharmacophore concepts in CADD (computer-aided drug design)

The pharmacophore concept has become an important tool in CADD. Each type of atom or group in a molecule that shows certain properties related to molecular identification can be reduced to a pharmacophore feature. These molecular patterns can be labelled as hydrogen bond donors or acceptors, cationic, anionic, aromatic, or hydrophobic, and any possible combinations. Different molecules can be compared at the pharmacophore level; this usage is often described as "pharmacophore finger-prints." When only a few pharmacophore features are considered in a 3D model the pharmacophore is sometimes described as a "query".

Pharmacophore Mapping/Modelling in Virtual Screening

Pharmacophore modelling is most frequently applied to virtual screening in order to recognize molecules triggering the desired biological effect. For this purpose, researchers generate a pharmacophore model (query) that most likely encodes the correct 3D organization of the required interaction pattern. Depending on how much is known about the particular protein target, different choices are available to build such a querys. Usually, it is good practice to separate the ligand data into two sets, training and an evaluation set to validate the generated pharmacophore query, when multiple active ligands (and inactive derivatives) are known (Fig. 7.2).

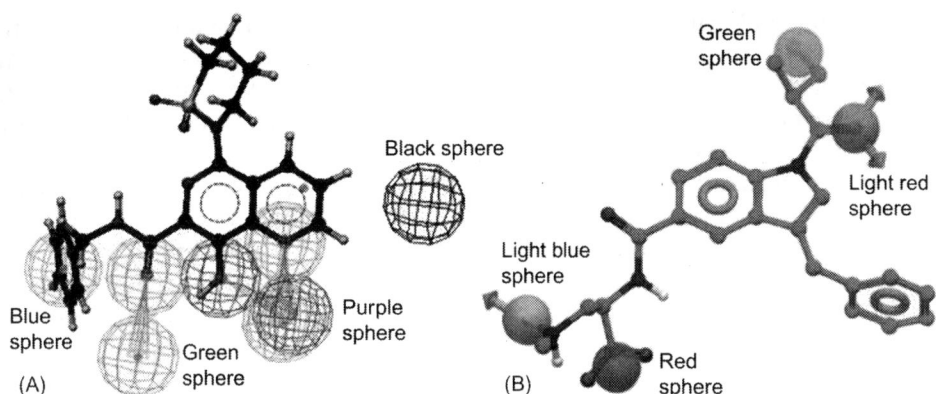

Fig. 7.2: Examples of pharmacophores used in ligand-based virtual screening **A.** A pharmacophore produced by catalyst. *Blue sphere*: Hydrophobic feature; *green sphere*: Hydrogen-bond acceptor; *purpl sphere*: Hydrogen-bond donor; *black sphere*: Excluded volume **B.** A pharmacophore produced by phase. *Light red sphere*: Hydrogen-bond acceptor; *light blue sphere*: Hydrogen-bond donor; *green sphere*: Hydrophobic feature; Red sphere: Negative feature; orange torus: Aromatic ring

No protein structure and no ligand structure is known: If the target structure and all its ligands are unknown, pharmacophore modeling is impossible. The only option to use the pharmacophore principle is to design a different library employing a metric based diversity on pharmacophore fingerprints to ensure optimal diversity of the library, containing a range of molecules with different pharmacophore feature composition. Certainly, considering the large number of available and potential compounds, the trend is to design libraries very carefully in order to cover chemical space efficiently in any search process.

No protein structure, but active ligand structures are known: The other situation is that the structure of the receptor (and any complex with the ligand) is unknown. This happens often in drug discovery. If only a single active molecule is known, then it is impossible to map the main contributing pharmacophore features onto the molecule, and the only choice may be to use similarity searches (such as using pharmacophore fingerprints) to recover similar molecules. Once these have been tested, a set of multiple active and inactive compounds may be known and more advanced pharmacophore modelling can be utilized.

Protein and ligand structures are known: In this case, structural information is available for both ligands and the receptor protein. Usually a pharmacophore model represents the main features of a small molecule that allow it to bind to some receptor molecule, but this idea can be reversed and pharmacophore queries built from features of a protein active site. These features describe the principle interactions between the protein and its ligands, and can be mapped onto the bioactive conformation of the ligand. Ideally the structural model is derived from crystallographic or nuclear magnetic resonance data, but homology models or other structural data can be used as well. Although a structure for one ligand may be enough, it is beneficial to have 3D information for multiple ligands to identify the common interactions. While this approach is compatible with the majority of pharmacophore modeling methods, LigandScout is the first software package able to construct automatically a query from one or more Protein Data Bank (PDB) files based on protein–ligand interactions.

Applications of pharmacophores in ADMET: Poor ADMET (pharmacokinetics and toxicity) is a key factor for failures during drug development and clinical trials. It is, therefore, widely accepted that the ADMET properties should be studied early during the drug discovery process, and pharmacophore modeling approaches are often used for such ADMET predictions. The pharmacophore models can be used to identify possible interactions of drugs with drug metabolizing enzymes by matching the equivalent chemical groups of test molecules to those of drug molecules with a well-known ADMET profile. The enzymes of major importance for observed ADMET profile are the cytochrome P450s (CYP) that initiate drug breakdown. It has been observed that only six CYP isoenzymes are responsible for over 90% of drug metabolism.

Limitations of Pharmacophore Methods

Despite the vast number of successful cases of drug designs relying on pharmacophore modeling, it is still not reliable and one should be cautious about the limitations of this technique:

1. The major limitation in virtual screening by pharmacophore is the absence of good scoring metrics. Whereas, docking simulations are based on scoring functions trying to calculate the binding affinity and similarity searches utilize similarity metrics such as the Tanimoto score, general scoring metric.
2. A second limitation is the dependency of a pharmacophore-based virtual screen on a pre-computed conformation database. These databases only contain a limited number of low-energy conformations per molecule.
3. Finally, a major limitation is that there is no proper method to construct a pharmacophore query.

8 | Chemoinformatics and Bioinformatics

CHEMOINFORMATICS

Modeling and informatics have become an indispensable components of rational drug design. Modeling in drug design has two facets:

a. modeling on the basis of knowledge of the drugs/leads/ligands and

b. modeling based on the structure of macromolecules.

The term chemoinfomatics also referred to as chemoinformatics or cheminformatics has been recognised in recent years as a distinct discipline in computational molecular sciences. Cheminformatics is also known as interface science as it combines physics, chemistry, biology, mathematics, biochemistry, statistics and informatics. It deals with discovering drugs based in modern drug discovery techniques which in turn rectifies complex issues in traditional drug discovery system. *Cheminformatics tools* help medicinal chemist for better understanding the complex structures of chemical compounds. Cheminformatics is emerging interdisciplinary field which primarily aims to discover Novel Chemical Entities (NCE) which ultimately results in design of new molecule (chemical data). It also plays an important role for collecting, storing and analysing the chemical data.

The primary focus of cheminformatics is to analyse/simulate/modelling/ manipulate chemical information which can be represented either in 2D structure or in 3D structure. Industry sectors such as, agrochemicals, food and pharmaceutical are distinct areas where cheminformatics plays significant role in the recent history of molecular sciences. It is the mixing of information resources to transform data into information and information into knowledge which is collectively referred as inductive learning. Cheminformatics has mainly dealt with small molecules, whereas bioinformatics addresses genes, proteins, and other larger chemical compounds. Chem and bioinformatics complements each other for bimolecular process, like structure and function of proteins, the binding of a ligand to its binding site, the conversion of a substrate within its enzyme receptor, and the catalysis of a biochemical reaction by an enzyme.

Different tools and methods are available to represent chemical structure, database to store chemical data, to perform searching process, quantitative structure–activity relationship (QSAR), quantitative structure–property relationship (QSPR), to predict physical, chemical and biological properties of a molecule.

The three areas of molecular informatics within pharmaceutical research— molecular modeling, cheminformatics, and bioinformatics act synergistically within drug design. Information feeds in all directions and the different areas interact differently with principal customers within the overall design and discovery process (as shown in Fig. 8.1).

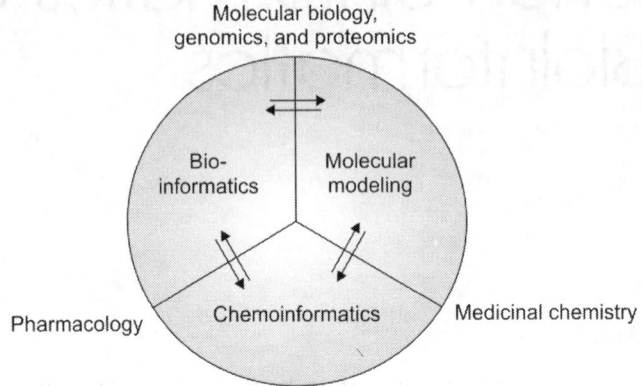

Fig 8.1: The synergy of molecular informatics

HOW IT WORKS

Most cheminformatics applications rely on large databases of chemical structures and their properties and relationships to, say, biological targets. Organizing and maintaining them, as well as searching and clustering similar structures all together, are essential for many scientic applications. However, each of these areas poses challenges to computer science; for example, chemical and bioactivity databases (such as ChEMBLdb and PubChem) are freely available and contain possibly millions (ChEM-BLdb) and tens of millions (PubChem) of data points. Integration of this completely different data is essential for researchers to gain the fullest possible perspective on what is presently known, tracking ongoing advances in science as they become available.The challenge for database search increases when considering protonation states (how the molecule changes when one proton is added to it) and tautomer states (how the molecule can change when a proton migrates from one part of the molecule to another). The need for a unique representation that is invariant with respect to atom ordering arises due to the expense of graph isomorphism (checking whether two structures represent the same molecule). Morgan described the structure as *unique representation algorithm*, or canonicalization algorithm, allowing chemists to generate unique string representations of chemical graphs and compare structures through string comparions. The simplied Molecular-Input Line-Entry System, or SMILES, format dened by Weininger in 1988is an example of a representation that can be canonicalized

NEED FOR CHEMINFORMATICS?

Cheminformatics plays a key role to maintain and access enormous amount of chemical data, produced by chemist (more than 45 million chemical compounds are known and the number may increase in million every year,) by using a proper database. Also, the field of chemistry needs a novel technique for knowledge extraction from data to model complex relationships between the structure of the chemical compound and biological activity or the influence of reaction condition on chemical reactivity. Cheminformatics has wider range of application.

Three major aspects of cheminformatics are:

i. Information acquisition, is a process of generating and collecting data empirically (experimentation) or from theory (molecular simulation)

ii. Information management deals with storage and retrieval of information and

iii. Information use, which includes data analysis, correlation, and application to problems in the chemical and biochemical sciences.

Applications of Cheminformatics

1. It is a significant application of information technology to help chemists for investigating new problems, organize, analyse, and understand scientific data in the development of novel compounds, materials and processes.

2. *Computer-Assisted Synthesis Design (CASD)* is applied mainly where artificial intelligence technique can be applied. This technique is applied in various applications which included pharmaceutical, food industry, textile industry and agro industry. Various forms of machine readable chemical representation play basic property to design chemical database where the chemical information are stored for analysis and manipulation. The chemical structure representations can be linear, 2D or in 3D format. SMILES (Simplified Molecular Input Line Entry Specification) is one of the linear chemical notation format which is widely used among chemist for various clinical and analysis purpose. Structure representation deals with Reaction Representation, Structure Descriptors, Molecular Modelling, Structure Searching, and Computer-Assisted Structure Elucidation (CASE).

2.1. Target identification and validation cheminformatics is used to identify target molecule which can be either gene or protein and could be a potential drug for the disease (Gene/Protein analysis). The identified protein is separated, crystallized and ligand binding processes are done. Some approaches will inhibit the disease functionality by making the key molecule stop functioning. Another approach is by promoting specific molecule in the normal way which may have affected in the disease state. These approaches and different databases can be applied for the discovery of drug targets. After target Identification, validation phase starts by determining whether the modulation of the target will yield a desired clinical outcome. This is based on the results obtained between the cellular location and disease/health condition, potential expression and protein binding state.

2.2. Lead identification: Target identification like protein, genes, hit phase high throughput screening (HTS) technique is applied where the protein targets are automatically screened against database of small-molecule or cell-based assay compounds. Lead identification also helps to see which molecules bind strongly to the target. Several similarity and diversity techniques can be applied for lead identification.

2.3. Lead optimization: This phase results in finding the drug candidate from the lead identified compound. The goal is a process of refining the chemical structure of a confirmed hit to improve its drug characteristics. Several docking techniques can be applied to optimize the lead structures for target affinity and selectivity. Different techniques and methods are used for Lead identification and Optimization process where some of the methods Virtual Screening, Molecular Database, Data mining, High-Throughput Screening (HTS), QSAR, Protein Ligand Models, Structure Based Models, Microarray analysis, Property Calculation and ADMET (adsorption, distribution, metabolism and elimination and toxicity).

Cheminformatics challenges: The key challenge for computational methods then is not traveling through chemical space per se, but rather to be able to focus traveling expeditions in a vast chemical space towards interesting regions, and to be able to recognize interesting stars and galaxies when they are encountered. The notion of what is interesting may vary of course with the task (e.g. drug discovery, reaction discovery, polymer discovery). But at the most fundamental level what is needed are tools to predict the physical, chemical, and biological properties of small molecules and reactions in order to focus searches and filter search results.

CONCLUSION

Cheminformatics, the computer science of chemical discovery, is an industrial and academic discipline with roots dating to the 19th century and a owering in the 1960s along with modern computing technologies. While many key cheminformatics techniques have been available in the literature since the 1960s, most cheminformatics tools and implementations have been proprietary; likewise, most data sources have been proprietary (usually with restrictive licensing policies) until recently. Companies look to protect their intellectual property for many reasons primarily involving prot, competitive intelligence, and intellectual property relevant to the pharmaceutical industry, as well as to other chemical-related industries. Unlike much of bio-informatics, these issues are where the data and tools have been freely available since the eld's inception. The disparity between cheminformatics and bioinformatics can be attributed to the fact that the outcomes from cheminformatics methods and software have a more direct effect on prots, in terms of identifying lead-like compounds and improving the properties of drug candidates, while bioinformatics soft-ware is found in upstream areas (such as target identication) and is perhaps less directly related to possible prots as a candidate small molecule. Moreover, acquiring chemical data (such as structure and activity) is more difcult and when done on a large scale can involve much time and effort, whereas acquiring bioinformatics data (such as sequences) is much easier.

Nevertheless, due to increasing availability of tools and data, the barrier to entry for non-chemists and non-cheminformaticians is signicantly lower than a decade ago. Many questions that would benet from computer science can now be addressed; for example, for theorists, graph-theoretic questions of 3D enumeration; for database designers, more effective search algorithms and ontologies; for practical programmers, expansion of the many open-source cheminformatics projects. If more chemists would think algorithmically and more computer scientists chemically, the pharmaceutical industry and associated industries would be much better positioned to deal with not only "simple" chemicals (only one identier and isomer possible per molecule) but also their complex relationships, transformations, and combinatorial challenges, bringing cheminformatics closer to the goal of supporting primary translational research in the wider context of chemical biology and systemchemistry.

BIOINFORMATICS

Bioinformatics, as a word if not as a discipline, has been around for about a decade, and as a word it tends to mean very different things in different contexts. Operating at the level of protein and nucleic acid primary sequences, it is a branch of information science handling medical, genomic and biological information to support of both clinical and more basic research. It deals with the similarity between macromolecular sequences, allowing for the identification of genes descended from a common ancestor, which share a corresponding structural and functional proximity.

Bioinformatics, as do most areas of science, relies on many other disciplines, both as a source of techniques and as a source of data. Bioinformatics also forms synergistic links with other areas of biology, most notably genomics, as both vendor and consumer. This is, by and large, concerned with data handling: the annotation of databases of macromolecular sequences and structures or the classification of sequences or structures into coherent groups. Prediction, as well as analysis, is also important, not least in trying to address two of the key challenges of the discipline: the prediction of function from sequence and the prediction of structure from sequence.Although these two are intimately linked, there is nonetheless still an important conceptual difference between them. One can discern three main areas within the traditional core of bioinformatics: one dealing with nucleic acid sequences, one with protein sequences, and one with macromolecular structures. With it, one can do so much: predict 3D structure, either through homology modelling or via de novo structure; identify functionally important residues; undertake phylogenetic analysis; and identify important motifs and thus develop discriminators for the membership of protein families. The definition of a protein family, the key step in annotating macromolecular sequences, proceeds through an iterative process of searching sequence, structure, and motif databases to generate a sequence corpus, which represents the whole set of sequences within the family. Motif databases, of which there are many, contain distilled descriptions of protein families that can be used to classify other sequences in an automated fashion. There are many ways to characterize motifs: through human inspection of sequence patterns, by using software to extract motifs from a multiple alignment, or using a program like MEME to generate motifs directly from a set of unaligned sequences. A motif or, more likely, a set of motifs defining the family can then be deposited in one of the many primary motif databases, such as PRINTS, or secondary, or derived, motif database, such as INTERPRO.

Data, Data Sets, and Annotations Limited catalogues of small molecules are available in digital format from many vendors across the world, as well as a number of public Web sites. As datasets of small molecules become increasingly available, it is important to develop computational methods to both organize these data in rapidly searchable databases and to extract or predict useful information for each molecule, including its physical, chemical, and biological properties. Conversely, large and well-annotated datasets are essential for developing statistical machine learning methods in cheminformatics, whether supervised or unsupervised, including predictive classification, regression, and clustering of small molecules and their properties. Aggregation and organization of datasets of chemical information allows for massive in silico processing that would be impractical or even impossible in a traditional experimental setting. Several parallel efforts have emerged recently to start to address the data bottleneck, including PubChem (http://pubchem.ncbi.nlm.nih.gov), the Harvard Chembank, UCSF's ZINC, and the UCI ChemDB. The UCI ChemDB is a public database containing over 4M compounds as well as a repository of annotated datasets that can be used to develop statistical machine learning methods. Together, these datasets already pose important challenges for both supervised and unsupervised machine learning methods, from clustering to kernel methods.

Within the pharmaceutical industry, and related areas, bioinformatics can be sub-divided into several complementary areas: gene informatics, protein informatics, and system informatics (Fig. 8.2). Gene informatics, links to genomics and MicroArray

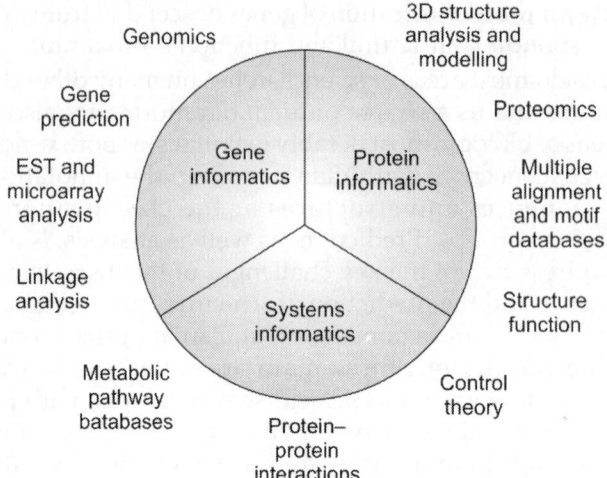

Fig. 8.2: The place of bioinformatics in pharmaceutical research

analysis, is concerned with managing information on genes and genomes and the in silico prediction of gene structure. Protein informatics concerns itself with managing information on protein sequences and has obvious links with proteomics and structure-function relationships. Part of its active area includes the modelling of 3D structure and the construction of multiple alignments. The third component concerns itself with the higher order interactions rather than simple sequences and includes the elaboration of functional protein–protein interactions, metabolic pathways, and control theory.

APPLICATIONS OF BIOINFORMATICS

This mechanism combines mathematics, statistics, and computer science and information technology to solve complex biological problems. These problems are generally the molecular level which cannot be solved by other means. This interesting field of science has many applications and research areas where it can be applied.

Sequence Analysis: The application of sequence analysis find outs those genes which encode regulatory sequences or peptides by using the information of sequencing. For sequence analysis, there are many powerful tools and computers which perform the duty of analyzing the genome of various organisms. These computers and tools also see the DNA mutations in an organism and also detect and identify those sequences which are related. Shotgun sequence techniques are also used for sequence analysis of numerous fragments of DNA. Special software is used to see the overlapping of fragments and their assembly.

Prediction of Protein Structure: It is easy to find out the primary structure of proteins in the form of amino acids which are present on the DNA molecule but it is hard to determine the secondary, tertiary or quaternary structures of proteins. For this purpose, either the method of crystallography is used or tools of bioinformatics can also be used to determine the complex protein structures.

Genome Annotation: In genome annotation, genomes are marked to know the regulatory sequences and protein coding. It is a very important part of the human genome project as it determines the regulatory sequences.

Comparative Genomics: Comparative genomics is the branch of bioinformatics which determines the genomic structure and function relation between different biological species. For this purpose, intergenomic maps are constructed to trace the processes of evolution that occur in genomes of different species. These maps contain the information about the point mutations as well as the information about the duplication of large chromosomal segments.

Health and Drug Discovery: The tools of bioinformatics are also helpful in drug discovery, diagnosis and disease management. Complete sequencing of human genes has allowed the scientists to make medicines and drugs which can target more than 500 genes. Different computational tools and drug targets has made the drug delivery simple and specific because now only those cells can be targeted which are diseased or mutated. It is also easy to know the molecular basis of a disease.

9

Database

INTRODUCTION

A database (DB), in the most general sense, is an organized collection of data. It is an electronic system that allows data to be easily accessed, manipulated and updated.

Many organization uses database as a method of storing, managing and retrieving information. Modern databases are managed using a database management system (DBMS).

Types of Databases

The different types database are:

1. Centralised
2. Operational
3. End-user
4. Commercial
5. Personal
6. Distributed

1. Centralised Database

Users from different locations can access this database from a remote location at the central database, that store entire information and application programs at a central computing facility for processing. The application programs pick up the appropriate data from the database based on the transactions sent by the communications controller for processing the transaction.

Data validation and verification is carried out by the application programs at the central computer centre, and a registration number is allotted by the application programs located at the central facility. The local area office keeps on recording it and hardly does any processing.

2. Operational Database

This is more of a basic form of data that contain information relating to the operations of an enterprise. Generally, such databases are organised on functional lines such as marketing, production, employees, *etc.*

3. End user Database

End user is the user of software, application or a product. This is a shared database which is shared by users and is meant for use by the end users, just like managers at different levels. They may not be concerned about the individual transactions as found in operational databases. This database is more about the summary of the information.

4. Commercial Database

This is a database that contains information which external users may require. However, they will not be able to afford maintaining such huge database by themselves. It's a paid service to the user as the databases are subject specific. The access to commercial database can be given through commercial links.

Some of the database service providers also offer databases on CD-ROMs and the updated versions of the databases are made available periodically. The databases on CD-ROMs have the advantage of reduced cost of communication.

5. Personal Database

The personal databases are maintained, generally, on personal computers. They contain information that is meant for use only among a limited number of users, generally working in the same department.

6. Distributed Database

These databases have contributions from the common databases as well as the data captured from the local operations. The data remains distributed at various sites in the organisation. As the sites are linked to each other with the help of communication links, the entire collection of data at all the sites constitutes the logical database of the organisation.

Types of Database as Applicable in Cheminformatics and Bioinformatics

1. ADME Database
2. Chemical Database
3. Biochemical Database
4. Drug/Pharmaceutical Database

1. ADME Database

Drug absorption, distribution, metabolism and excretion (ADME) habitually involve interaction of a drug with particular ligands/proteins. Information about these ADME-linked proteins is essential in facilitating the study of the molecular mechanism of disposition and individual response as well as therapeutic action of drugs. It is also useful in the progress and testing of pharmacokinetics prediction tools

ADME Database also contains the updated and comprehensive data on interactions of substances with Drug Metabolizing Enzymes and Drug Transporters. It is intended for use in drug research and development, including drug–drug interactions and ADME (Absorption, Distribution, Metabolism and Excretion) studies. The information is provided by category (therapeutic area), drug name, enzyme, reaction, and type. It is supported by chemical/metabolite structures as well as kinetic values mentioned in the literature (Fig. 9.1). The contents of the database were collected and organized according to the original Human P_{450} and Transporter Metabolism Database. The database is accessible online and completely searchable by keywords or chemical structures. Advanced searches are also obtainable to support investigational studies on drug-drug interactions. ADME Database contains more than 26,000 substances, several natural products and preparations, in addition to other factors effecting Drug Metabolizing Enzymes activity. The data collected from more than 18,000 citations.

Features of human drug metabolizing enzyme databases: It contains information on CYP enzymes (Cytochrome P450) and a number of variants, which are tested in the metabolism of xenobiotics and endobiotics in humans. It provides information on substances (as well as a number of natural products and other factors) influencing CYP activity based on the interactions with substrate, inhibitor, inducer and activator.

The database gives other enzymes information also such as Esterases, UDP-glucuronosyl transferases, Sulphotransferases, Glutathione S-transferases, Flavin-containing Monooxygenases.

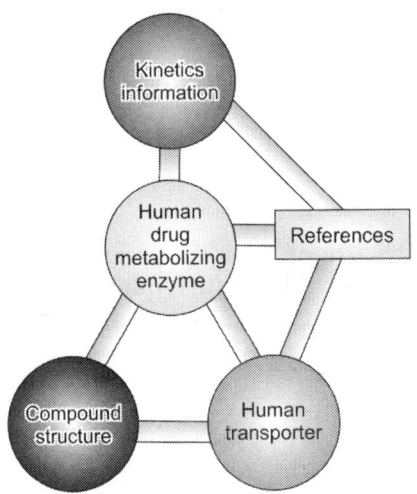

Fig. 9.1: ADME database

Kinetics information database: It contains supporting entries for the Human Drug Metabolizing Enzyme Database, providing numerical data on major kinetic parameters relevant for use in drug development/application studies. It provides information about *in vitro* assay used, K_m, V_{max}, K_i, K_inactivation, Cooperativityn), IC_{50}, EC_{50}, $t_{1/2}$ The kinetic database is accessible only when it is joined with Human Drug Metabolizing Enzyme Database.

Human drug transporter database: It contains information on transporters involved in transport of drugs, physiological compounds, nutrients, and other chemicals and metabolites. It is featured with ABC Transporters, Organic Ion Transporters, Peptide Transporters, Nucleotide Transporters, *etc.*

Apart from above mentioned database, a number of databases describing specific classes of ADME-associated proteins have appeared. A new database, ADME-associated proteins (ADME-AP), is introduced to give complete information about all classes of ADME-associated proteins illustrated in the literature including physiological function of each ligang/protein, ADME classification, pharmacokinetic effect, direction and driving force of disposition, location and tissue distribution, synonyms, substrates, gene name and protein availability in other species. Cross-links to other databases are also provided to help the access of information about the sequence, function, 3D structure, genetic disorders, polymorphisms, nomenclature, ligand binding properties and related literatures of each protein. ADME-AP at present has entries for 321 proteins and 964 substrates.

2. Chemical Database

A chemical database is a database specially designed to store chemical information. It contains information about chemical such as crystal structures, spectra, synthesis, reactions and thermophysical data. Chemical databases are the backbone of computer-aided drug discovery, whether it is chemoinformatics or bioinformatics. These databases provide information which can be used to build knowledge-based models for discovering and designing drug molecules.

Types of chemical databases:

i. **Chemical structure database:** Chemical structures are usually represented using lines indicating chemical bonds between atoms and 2D structure drawn on paper. They may be perfect visual representations for the chemist, but they are inappropriate for computational use and particularly for search and storage. Small molecules or ligands, are usually represented using lists of atoms and their connections. Large molecules such as proteins are however more efficiently represented using the sequences of their amino acid building blocks. Large chemical databases for structures are expected to handle the storage and searching of information on millions of molecules taking terabytes of physical memory.

Chemical structures are represented by two principal techniques:
- As connection tables/adjacency matrices/lists with additional information on bond (edges) and atom attributes (nodes), such as: MDL Molfile, CML, PDB
- As a linear string notation based on depth first or breadth first traversal, such as: SLN, WLN, SMILES/SMARTS, InChI

These approaches have been developed to permit representation of stereo-chemical differences and charges as well as special types of bonding such as those present in organo-metallic compounds. The main advantage of a computer representation is the possibility for increased storage and fast, flexible search.

ii. **Literature database:** Chemical literature databases correlate structures or other chemical information to significant references such as research papers or patents. This type of database includes Scifinder, STN and Reaxys. Links to literature are also present in many databases that focus on chemical characterization.

iii. **Crystallographic database:** Contains X-ray crystal structure data. Common examples include Protein Data Bank and Cambridge Structural Database.

iv. **NMR spectra database:** Associates chemical structure with NMR data. These databases often contain other characterization data such as FTIR and mass spectrometry.

v. **Reactions database:** Most chemical databases contain information on stable molecules but in databases for reactions, intermediates and temporarily created unstable molecules are also present. Reaction databases contain information about products, educts, and reaction mechanisms.

vi. **Thermophysical database:** Contains information about phase equilibria including solubility of gases in liquids, vapor–liquid equilibrium, liquids in solids (SLE), vaporization, heats of mixing, and fusion. It also stores caloric data like heat of formation, heat capacity, combustion, and transport properties such as viscosity and thermal conductivity

Various free databases available for chemical structure search are enlisted here:

PubChem: It was, released in 2004, gives information on the biological activities of small molecules. PubChem is organized as three linked databases within the NCBI's Entrezinformation retrieval system. These are PubChem Substance, PubChem Compound, and PubChem BioAssay. PubChem also provides a fast chemical structure similarity search tool. More information about using each component database may be found using the links in the homepage.

Links from PubChem's chemical structure records to other Entrez databases provide information on biological properties.

ChemSpider: It is a free chemical structure database providing fast text and structure search access to over 28 million structures from hundreds of data sources.

ChemFrog: ChemFrog is a chemical database that offers over 1 million commercially available chemicals and vendor information.

ChemDB: ChemDB is the IGB Chemical Database: The most diverse and useful set of chemoinformatics tools and applications existing for the public.

Applications: Chemical Search Finds a chemical by basic criteria like molecular weight and predicted log P, or by the additional abstract notion of structural similarity.

Virtual Chemical Space Interactively deconstructs target compounds into component precursors and reconstructs similar building-blocks into combinatorial libraries representing the "virtual chemical space" near the target compound.

Reaction ExplorerInteractive system for learning and practicing reactions, syntheses and mechanisms in organic chemistry, with advanced support for the automatic generation of random problems, curved-arrow mechanism diagrams, and inquiry-based learning.

COSMOS Predicts 3D small molecule structures from various standard 2D formats. Reaction Predictor predicts Mechanistic Reactions Using Machine Learning

iScienceSearch: It is an internet search engine used by chemists. iScienceSearch also supports mobile devices and it works well to draw structures on something like an iPad.

Chemicalize (www.chemicalize.org) from ChemAxon calculates structure parameters.

The DistilBio (a powerful, federated, life sciences search engine) new release now has instant display of results at http://www. distilbio.com with instantaneous search results and auto-complete, it is now even easier to find the research you are looking for all in one place. Visit the site and try it with "Aspirin".

3. Biochemical Database

The biology and biochemistry research communities have long recognised the need for the creation of database systems to support their research activities. This credit is encouraged by the ever-growing amount of biochemical data, generated by the use of new high-throughput experimental technologies and methods. Already, the analysis of biological data using traditional database systems is leading to the discovery of new relationships among concepts, the definition of new experiments, the creation of new methods and the isolation and definition of new concepts, though there is still a lot to do to develop data integration, representation and understanding. Researchers need a sophisticated access to this wealth of biochemical and biological data, a demand that traditional data management techniques struggle to meet. A biochemical database system needs to support research and scientific activities, helping in the formulation of hypotheses which are subsequently to be corroborated or falsified by experiments.

Biochemical pathways are subject to deep experimental research due to their role in cell metabolism. Thus, when designing a system to support their modelling and analysis it is necessary to consider the rapid growth of concepts and relations being represented in the database model.

Data associated with biochemical pathways is stored in many data repositories, with different access mechanisms, formats and structures. In order to make sense of these data it is compulsory to integrate them in a broad manner. Some biochemical databases are listed here:

- **Pathguide:** It contains information about 231 biological pathway resources. Click on a link to go to the resource home page or 'Details' for a description page.

- **BioCarta:** Observe how genes interact in dynamic graphical models. It also catalogs and summarizes important resources providing information for over 120,000 genes from multiple species.

- **BioSilico** is a web-based database system that facilitates the search and analysis of metabolic pathways. Heterogeneous metabolic databases including **ENZYME**, **LIGAND**, **EcoCyc** and **MetaCyc** are integrated in a systematic way, thereby allowing users to efficiently retrieve the relevant information on enzymes, biochemical compounds and reactions.

- **The Human Cancer Protein Interaction Network (HCPIN)** is a web-accessible database. It is designed for use by cancer biologists interested in assessing 3D protein structural information in the context of the protein interaction network."

- **KEGG** is a database of biological systems, consisting of genetic building blocks of genes and proteins (KEGG GENES), chemical building blocks of both endogenous and exogenous substances (KEGG LIGAND), molecular wiring diagrams of interaction and reaction networks (KEGG PATHWAY), and hierarchies and relationships of various biological objects (KEGG BRITE). KEGG provides a reference knowledge base for linking genomes to biological systems and also to environments by the processes of PATHWAY mapping and BRITE mapping."

- **STRING** is a database, provides information about known and predicted protein-protein interactions.

     The interactions contain direct (physical) and indirect (functional) associations; they are derived from four sources like High-throughput Experiments, Genomic Context, Coexpression and Previous Knowledge

- **Unified Human Interactome** is a broad database of the computational and experimental based human protein interaction networks. This database is aimed to incorporate diverge maps, which presents the research a flexible and direct entry gate into the human interactome. In its first version, it contains more than 178,000 different interactions between over 18,500 unique human proteins.

- **BRENDA:** Data on enzyme function are extracted directly from the primary literature by scientists holding a degree in Biology or Chemistry. Formal and consistency checks are done by computer programs, each data set on a classified enzyme is checked manually by at least one biologist and one chemist.

4. Drug Databases

Drug database provides information about chemical, pharmacodynamic, pharmacokinetic property details of the drug. It is essential in bioinformatics and cheminformatics studies to find most efficient and safe drug. Some of the drug databases are discussed here:

i. **DrugBank:** It is a unique bioinformatics and cheminformatics resource. It contains extensive data on the nomenclature, ontology, chemistry, structure, function, action, pharmacology, pharmacokinetics, metabolism and pharmaceutical properties of both small molecule and large molecule drugs. The database contains nearly 4300 drug entries including >1,000 FDA-approved small molecule drugs, 113 FDA-approved biotech (protein/peptide) drugs, 62 nutraceuticals and >3,000 experimental drugs. Additionally, more than 6,000 protein (i.e. drug target) sequences are linked to these drug entries. Each DrugCard entry contains more than 80 data fields with half of the information being devoted to drug/chemical data and the other half devoted to drug target or protein data. Table 9.1 shows the amount of information available in DrugBank has increased considerably since the first version.

Table 9.1: Comparison between the coverage in DrugBank 1.0, 2.0 and DrugBank 3.0 versions

Version	1.0	2.0	3.0
No. of data fields	88	108	148
No. of search types	8	12	16
No. of drug-action pathways	0	0	223
No. of drugs with metabolizing enzyme data	0	0	762
No. of drug metabolites	0	0	811
No. of drugs with drug transporter data	0	0	516
No. of SNP-associated drug effects	0	0	113
No. of drugs with patent/pricing/manufacturer data	0	0	1208
No. of food–drug interactions	0	714	1039
No. of drug–drug interactions	0	13242	13795
No. of ADMET parameters (Caco-2, LogS)	0	276	890
No. of QSAR parameters per drug	5	6	14
No. of FDA-approved small molecule drugs	841	1344	1424
No. of biotech drugs	113	123	132
No. of nutraceutical drugs	61	69	82
No. of withdrawn drugs	0	57	68

(Contd.)

Table 9.1: Comparison between the coverage in DrugBank 1.0, 2.0 and DrugBank 3.0 versions

Version	1.0	2.0	3.0
No. of illicit drugs	0	188	189
No. of experimental drugs	2894	3116	5210
Total No. of experimental and FDA small molecule drugs	3796	4774	6684
Total No. of experimental and FDA drugs	3909	4897	6816
No. of names/brands/synonyms	18304	28447	37171
No. of approved-drug drug targets (unique)	524	1565	1768
No. of all drug targets (unique)	2133	3037	4326
No. of approved-drug enzymes/carriers (unique)	0	0	164
No. of all drug enzymes/carriers (unique)	0	0	169
No. of external database links	12	18	31

ii. **Drugs.com** is the most trendy, broad and updated source of drug information online. It provides free, correct and independent guidance on more than 24,000 prescription drugs, over-the-counter medicines and natural products.

iii. **PharmGKB** provides information that establishes knowledge about the relationships between drugs, diseases and genes, including their differences and gene products.

10 | Molecular Mechanics and Quantum Mechanics

INTRODUCTION

Molecular mechanics, also called classical mechanics, explains molecules in terms of *bonded atoms*, which have been distorted from some idealized geometry due to non-bonded Coulombic and van der Waals interactions. This is primarily different from quantum chemical models, which is not related to chemical bonding. The achievement of molecular mechanics model depends on the high level of transferability of geometrical parameters from one molecule to another, as well as reliance of the parameters on atomic hybridization. For example, carbon-carbon single bond lengths usually fall in the small range from 1.45 to 1.55 Å, and increase in length with increasing *p-character* of the carbon hybrids. Thus, it is possible to provide a quite exact *guess* at molecular geometry in terms of bond angles, bond lengths and torsion angles, provided that the particular molecule has known valence structure. The bulk of organic molecules come into this category.

The quantum mechanics (QM) method considers molecules as collections of electrons and nuclei without any concern with *chemical bonds*. QM method understands the behaviour of systems at the atomic level. QM methods use the laws of QM to estimate the wave function and to solve the Schrödinger equation (it is a mathematical equation that explains the change over time of a physical system in which quantum effects such as wave function, are significant). The result to the Schrödinger equation is in terms of the movements of electrons, which consecutively lead to molecular structure and energy among other observables, as well as to information about bonding. According to QM, an electron bound to an atom cannot possess any arbitrary energy or occupy any position in space.

Although, study of interactions between proteins and ligands by QM methods is not a new approach in computational chemistry, it has been gaining popularity in the recent years. QM methods conquer the deficiencies of conventional force-field scoring functions by neglecting atom type assignment and parameterization. For a system, with distinct positions of the nuclei, they provide a dependable base for ligand geometry and energy estimations.

Molecular Mechanics

In the molecular mechanics, *energy* of a molecule is described as a sum of contributions arising from alterations from *ideal* bond angles (bend contributions), bond distances (stretch contributions), and torsion angles (torsion contributions), jointly with contributions due to *non bonded* (van der Waals and Coulombic) interactions. It is generally referred to *strain energy*, which reflects the *strain* inherent to a *real* molecule.

$$E^{\text{strain}} = E_A{}^{\text{stretch}} + E_A{}^{\text{bend}} + E_A{}^{\text{torsion}} + E_{AB}{}^{\text{Non-bonded}} \tag{10.1}$$

The first three summations in Eq. (10.1) are over all *bonds*, all *bond angles* and all *torsion angles*, respectively. Hence, information about bonding is *part of the input* to a molecular mechanics calculation, in contrast to a quantum chemical calculation where it is *part of the output*. The last summation in Eq. (10.1) is over all pairs of atoms which are not bonded.

Stretch and bend terms are most simply given in terms of quadratic (*Hook's law*) forms.

$$E^{\text{stretch}} (r) = \frac{1}{2} \, k^{\text{stretch}} \, (r - r^{\text{eq}})^2 \tag{10.2}$$

$$E^{\text{bend}} (\alpha) = \frac{1}{2} k^{\text{bend}} (\alpha - \alpha^{\text{eq}})^2 \tag{10.3}$$

r and α are the bond distance and angle, respectively, r^{eq} and α^{eq} are the *ideal* (equilibrium) bond length and bond angle, respectively, taken either from experiment or from accurate quantum chemical calculations, and k^{stretch} and k^{bend}, so-called stretch and bend *force constants*, respectively, are parameters. Molecular mechanics models may also contain cubic or higher-order contributions, as well as *cross terms* to account for correlations between stretch and bend components. The level of complexity depends on the availability of data on which to base parameters. Proper explanation of the torsional potential needs a form that reflects its inherent periodicity. For example, the three-fold periodicity of rotation about the carbon-carbon bond in ethane may be described by the simple functional form.

$$E^{\text{torsion}} (\omega) = k^{\text{torsion3}} \, [1 - \cos 3 \, (\omega - \omega^{\text{eq}})] \tag{10.4}$$

ω is the torsion angle, ω^{eq} is the ideal torsion angle and k^{torsion3} is treated as a parameter. Bond torsion contributions to the overall energy may also need to include terms which are one-fold and two-fold periodic.

$$E^{\text{torsion}} (\omega) = k^{\text{torsion1}} \, [1 - \cos (\omega - \omega^{\text{eq}})] + k^{\text{torsion2}} \, [1 - \cos 2 \, (\omega - \omega^{\text{eq}})] + k^{\text{torsion3}} \, [1 - \cos 3 \, (\omega - \omega_{\text{eq}})] \tag{10.5}$$

k^{torsion1}, k^{torsion2} and k^{torsion3} are additional parameters. Equation (10.5) is a truncated Fourier series. The one-fold term accounts for the difference in energy between *cis* ($0°$) and *trans* ($180°$) conformers, and the two-fold term accounts for the difference in energy between planar ($0°$, $180°$) and perpendicular ($90°$, $270°$) conformers. Molecular mechanics models may also consist of higher-order terms and cross terms, as well as terms to account for asymmetrical environments. As with stretch and bend components, the level of complexity depends on the availability of data on which to base parameters. Non-bonded interactions normally occupy a sum of van der Waals (VDW) interactions and Coulombic interactions.

$$E^{\text{non-bonded}} (r) = E^{\text{VDW}} (r) + E^{\text{Coulombic}} (r) \tag{10.6}$$

Additional non-bonded terms may be involved to find out interactions such as hydrogen bonding. Preferably, van der Waals interactions are considered as a sum of repulsive and attractive forces.

$$E^{VDW}(r) = \varepsilon[\,(r^0/r)^{12} - 2\,(r^0/r)^6\,] \tag{10.7}$$

where, r is the non-bonded distance, ε and r^0 are parameters. This functional form offers a very steep energy barrier inside the sum of van der Waals radii for the two atoms involved. This equation is used calculate both the inherent size requirements of atoms, as well as the weak attractive forces between separated atoms.

The Coulombic term is used to calculate the interaction of charges.

$$E^{Coulombic}(r) = \frac{qq'}{2} \tag{10.8}$$

r is the non-bonded distance, and the atomic charges q, may either be treated as parameters or be taken from quantum chemical calculations. The sum of atomic charges needs to be equal the total molecular charge, 0 in the case of a neutral molecule.

Applications of Molecular Mechanics

The main use of molecular mechanics is in the field of molecular dynamics. This uses the force fields such as SYBYL, MMFF to calculate the forces acting on each particle and a suitable integrator to model the dynamics of the particles and predict trajectories. The molecular dynamics trajectories can be used to estimate thermodynamic parameters of a system or probe kinetic properties, such as reaction rates and mechanisms.

Another application of molecular mechanics is energy minimization, whereby the force field is used as an optimization measure. This method uses a suitable algorithm (e.g. steepest descent) to find the molecular structure of a local energy minimum. These minima correspond to stable conformers of the molecule (in the chosen force field) and molecular motion can be modelled as vibrations around and interconversions between these stable conformers. It is thus common to find local energy minimization methods combined with global energy optimization, to find the global energy minimum (and other low energy states). At finite temperature, the molecule spends most of its time in these low-lying states, which thus dominate the molecular properties. Global optimization can be accomplished using simulated annealing, the Metropolis algorithm and Monte carlo methods, or using different deterministic methods of discrete or continuous optimization. While the force field characterizes only the enthalpic component of free energy (and only this component is included during energy minimization), it is possible to incorporate the entropic component through the use of additional methods, such as normal mode analysis.

Molecular mechanics potential energy functions have been used to determine binding constants, protein folding kinetics, protonation equilibria, active site coordinates, and to design binding sites.

Limitations of Molecular Mechanics Models

There are important limitations of molecular mechanics models. First, they are limited to the description of equilibrium geometries and equilibrium conformations. Because the mechanics *strain energy* is specific to a given molecule, strain energies cannot be used in thermochemical calculations. Two main exceptions are calculations concerning isomers with exactly the same bonding, e.g. comparison of *cis* and *trans*-2-butene, and conformational energy comparisons, where different conformers essentially have exactly the similar bonding. *Second*, molecular mechanics calculations disclose nothing about bonding or, more usually, about electron distributions in molecules. Third, presently available force fields have not been parameterized to hold non-equilibrium forms, particularly in reaction transition states. Note, however, that there is no fundamental reason why this could not be done (using results from quantum chemical calculations rather than experiment as a basis for parameterization). Finally, it requires to be noted that molecular mechanics is fundamentally an interpolation method, the success of which depends not only on good parameters, although also on systematics among related molecules. Molecular mechanics models would not be expected to be very successful in describing the structures and conformations of *new* (unfamiliar) molecules outside the range of parameterization.

Quantum Mechanics (QM)

QM describes the properties of molecules and atoms and their constituents such as electrons, protons, neutrons. These properties consist of the interactions of the particles with one another and with electromagnetic radiations like light, X-rays, and gamma rays.

The performance of matter and radiation on the atomic level frequently seems odd, and the consequences of quantum theory are therefore not easy to understand and to judge. The study of quantum mechanics is important for many reasons. First, it demonstrates the vital methodology of physics. Second, it has been extremely successful in giving accurate results in every situation to which it has been applied. An important feature of quantum mechanics is that it is normally impossible to measure a system without disturbing it; the thorough nature of this disturbance and the correct point at which it occurs are unclear and controversial. Hence, quantum mechanics attracted scientists of the 20th century to get the finest intellectual construction of the period.

Basic Concept of Quantum Mechanics

After Bohr's theory, which assumed that electrons moved in circular orbits, QM fundamentally based upon two approaches: (a) matrix mechanics, proposed by Werner Heisenberg and (b) wave mechanics given by Erwin Schrödinger. The present conversation follows Schrödinger's wave mechanics because it is less abstract and easier to understand than Heisenberg's matrix mechanics.

Schrödinger's Wave Mechanics

Schrödinger articulated de Broglie's hypothesis about the wave behaviour of matter in a mathematical equation that is flexible to a variety of physical troubles without additional arbitrary assumptions. He referred to a mathematical formulation of optics, in which the straight-line propagation of light rays can be derived from wave motion when the wavelength is small compared to the dimensions of the apparatus employed. Similarly, Schrödinger find a wave equation for matter that would give particle-like propagation when the wavelength becomes comparatively small. According to conventional mechanics, if a particle of mass m_e is subjected to a force such that its potential energy is $V(x, y, z)$ at position x, y, z, then the sum of $V(x, y, z)$ and the kinetic energy $p^2/2m_e$ is equal to a constant, the total energy E of the particle.

Thus,

$$\frac{p^2}{2m_e} + V(x, y, z) = E \qquad (10.9)$$

It is believed that the particle is bound, restricted by the potential to a particular region in space because its energy E is insufficient for it to escape. Since the potential changes with position, two other things, the momentum and the wavelength of the wave would also change. Assuming a wave function $\Psi(x, y, z)$ that varies with position, Schrödinger replaced p *(momentum)* in the above energy equation with a differential operator. He then showed that Ψ satisfies the partial differential equation

$$-\frac{h^2}{2m_e}\left(\frac{\delta^2\psi}{\delta x^2} + \frac{\delta^2\psi}{\delta x^2} + \frac{\delta^2\psi}{\delta x^2}\right) + V(x, y, z)\,\psi = E\psi \qquad (10.10)$$

This is the (time-independent) Schrödinger wave equation, which recognized quantum mechanics in a broadly applicable form. A significant advantage of Schrödinger's theory is that no further arbitrary quantum conditions need be postulated. The required quantum results follow from certain reasonable restrictions placed on the wave function—for example, that it should not become infinitely large at large distances from the centre of the potential.

The Schrödinger equation cannot be solved accurately for atoms with more than one electron. The principles of the calculation are well known, but the problems are complicated by the number of particles and the range of forces involved. The forces consist of the electrostatic forces between the nucleus and the electrons and between the electrons themselves, as well as weaker magnetic forces arising from the spin and orbital motions of the electrons. These problems resolved by approximation methods, assuming that each electron moves independently in an average electric field because of the nucleus and the other electrons, i.e. correlations between the positions of the electrons are neglected. Each electron has its own wave function, called an orbital. The overall wave function for all the electrons in the atom satisfies the exclusion principle. Corrections to the calculated energies are then made, which depend on the strengths of the electron-electron correlations and the magnetic forces.

Applications of Quantum Mechanics Drug Discovery

The application of QM based approaches in structure based drug designing is not new. QM has been applied to some medicinally relevant chemistry calculations for providing informative descriptors for QSAR and 3D conformation for ligands. Quantum mechanics methods are able to provide an accurate representation of ligands and proteins where molecular mechanics parameterization struggles. QM mechanics approaches hold promise in addressing pharmacological problems on the time scale demanded by drug-discovery research.

The use of QM-Molecular mechanics approaches in computation of protein–ligand binding affinities has found mixed success. Though, the Quantum mechanics-Molecular mechanics approach seems to be beneficial for low-resolution X-ray structures, where an inaccurate ligand structure is available. Study tells that the use of accurate charges, in several cases, leads to development in docking accuracy in a wide range of Protein Data Bank complexes.

Typical applications of QM in drug design involve the calculation of energies and structure optimization of ligand and/or protein–ligand complexes, particularly for docking studies to get the correct binding mode of a ligand. Quantum mechanics-Molecular mechanics methods have shown accurate results when employed in the calculation of binding energies. Though, this approach still needs further sampling of ligand–target conformations through molecular dynamics simulations. QM methods have proved useful in the study of some target proteins, including HIV1 integrase, trypsin, West Nile virus NS3 serine protease, HIV1PR, and CDK2.

Quantum mechanics method used to replicate an experimental work accurately, offers a potential solution to the failures mentioned. Another development in drug design research is the hybrid Quantum mechanics-Molecular mechanics method, developed to improve the accuracy of biomolecular simulations, Quantum mechanics docking, Quantum mechanics virtual screening, and Quantum mechanics-QSAR. The quantum mechanics approach has been successfully applied in drug discovery in pharmaceutical companies, e.g. in the combination of artificial intelligence and cloud computing to search molecular entities and aid in the design of novel drugs.

The QM is not limited to computational model of a drug only, it can also be applied to proteins, DNA, carbohydrates, and lipids, as well as solvent molecules that are involved in drug transportation, binding, and signalling.

QM IMPLEMENTATION IN THE PHARMACEUTICAL INDUSTRY: TIME VS ACCURACY

As the ADMET properties of a drug decide its activity, the development of a new drug with reasonable ADMET makes drug discovery a more difficult and challenging process in the pharmaceutical industry. The pharmaceutical industry is gradually operating in an era where development costs are continuously under pressure, higher percentages of drugs are demanded, and the drug-discovery is a trial-and-error run process.

In recent years, the use of computer-aided drug designing to simulate drug–receptor interactions has made drug designing realistic, reasonable and cost-effective. *In silico* tools, such as docking, virtual screening, QSAR, molecular simulation, molecular mechanics, and quantum mechanics, use their respective mathematical equation to predict quickly the binding affinities of a large library of compounds, as well as analyze homolytic or heterolytic fission/fusion before undergoing chemical (synthesis) and biological (activity) evaluation as a novel compound. Compared to those used in pharmaceutical companies, there are more efficient methods, but the cost with respect to computer time/resources is high when one has to scan a really large library of compounds. Therefore, using a combination of quantum mechanics to parameterize the molecules and molecular mechanics to explain and solvate the protein, a more precise understanding of binding affinity and protein–molecule interaction could be achieved (Fig. 10.1). This method implemented in pharmaceutical companies' R&D to achieve correct binding affinities and free binding energy using different ligand geometries in Quantum mechanics–Molecular mechanics energy calculations. Furthermore, using QSAR to predict the activity of an existent molecule may lead to remarkable savings with respect to development time and cost.

Abbreviations: ADMET, absorption, distribution, metabolism, excretion, toxicity; QM, quantum mechanics.

Perhaps, most pharmaceutical companies today follow common technology processes for discovering drugs. These consist of cloning and expression of human receptors and enzymes using high-throughput, automated screening and the application of combinatorial chemistry. The field of combinatorial chemistry is in constant progress.

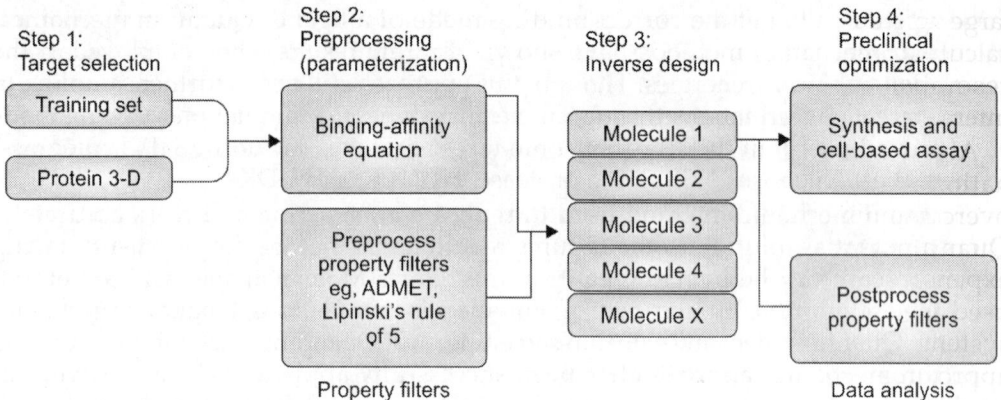

Fig.10.1: Implementation of QM in pharmaceutical companies' drug design workflow

Molecular Mechanics or Quantum Mechanics—Which to Choose?

Classical mechanics, also called molecular mechanics, is the alternative to quantum mechanics when chemical reactions do not need to be considered in a simulation. Molecular mechanics does not start from an *exact theory* (the Schrödinger equation), but rather describes molecules in terms of *bonded atoms*, which have been distorted from some idealized geometry due to unbound van der Waals and Columbic interactions. Though molecular mechanics does not solve the Schrödinger equation for electron motions, it requires an explicit description of chemical bonding and lots of information about the structures of molecules. It is the use and extent of this information that distinguishes different Molecular mechanics models. While many of the details of mechanical and biochemical interactions in enzymes are currently unclear, molecular mechanics can rely on force fields with fixed parameters to provide better understanding of conformational analysis between conformers, mechanical deformation of DNA, RNA, and proteins, and changes in cellular structure, response, and function. This understanding can offer new prognoses of diseases, as molecular mechanics calculations are used to provide qualitative descriptions of molecular interactions.

Quantum mechanics has been said to succeed outstandingly in the area where molecular mechanics failed. In contrast to quantum mechanics, molecular mechanics ignores electrons, fails to illustrate reality, and also computes the energy of a system as only a function of the nuclear positions. Generally, QM incorporates four phenomena for which molecular mechanics cannot justify. These include quantization of some physical properties, quantum entanglement, the principle of uncertainty, and wave–particle duality. Quantum mechanics is applied in the determination of interactions between possible drugs and enzyme active sites. It is slow but accurate with respect to drug designing. In spite of the advantages of molecular mechanics, it has some setbacks, such as inappropriate parameterization, inability to predict chemical reactions, or explain bond breaking/formation.

Quantum Mechanics–Molecular Mechanics Hybrid in Computer-Aided Drug Designing (CADD)

The computational chemists have a huge selection of methodologies for designing a new drug. The key tools available belong to six all-encompassing classes: Molecular dynamic simulation, molecular mechanics, quantum mechanics, *ab initio* calculations, DFT, and semiempirical calculations. Molecular mechanics can be used to study very large molecules, because other Quantum mechanics methods, such as semiempirical calculations, *ab initio*, and DFT are relatively slow and would exhaust computational resources. However, Molecular mechanics methods are unable to deal with interactions between the ligand and the receptor in metal-containing systems.

Algorithms such as hybrid quantum mechanics/molecular mechanics, a combination of quantum mechanics and molecular mechanics have been developed to overcome the limitations brought by the individual application of these methods. Quantum mechanics methods are the most accurate, but also computationally expensive and time-consuming calculations. Quantum mechanics calculations are used in semiempirical methods (e.g. AM1, PM3) only for valence electrons in the system, whereas for other electrons and atomic nuclei behavior of other atoms, approximations are required. Combined quantum mechanics–molecular mechanics methods provide the precision of a quantum mechanics description with low computational cost of molecular mechanics. Even though quantum mechanics-Molecular mechanics may not be applicable in every structure based drug designing project, but the majority of assignments can be well addressed by this hybrid method. Quantum mechanics–molecular mechanics is thus the crucial component in computational drug discovery.

Five key facets are crucial in planning a Quantum mechanics-Molecular mechanics calculation on an enzyme: choice of the Quantum mechanics method, choice of molecular mechanics force field, segregation of the system into Quantum mechanics and molecular mechanics regions, simulation type (e.g. Molecular dynamics simulation or calculation of potential energy profiles), and whether advanced conformational sampling will be performed. The choice of Quantum mechanics method is crucial. A variety of different Quantum mechanics methods is available, ranging from fast, semiempirical methods (e.g. AM1, PM3, SCC-DFTB; low accuracy and maximum of 2,000 atoms) to more accurate but more computationally expensive Hartree–Fock and density-functional (e.g. B3LYP; medium accuracy and maximum of 500 atoms), and molecular orbital ab initio (e.g. MP2, coupled cluster; very high accuracy and maximum of 20 atoms) methods. Not all methods are applicable to all systems, for reasons of accuracy, practicality, or lack of parameters (e.g. for semiempirical methods) (Table 10.1). Generally, but not always, improved accuracy comes at the price of increased calculation expenses.

Progressively more, Quantum mechanics–molecular mechanics methods are being applied to enzymes that are drug targets, often with the aim of providing information for drug designing. Examples include the HIV1-replication enzymes: reverse transcriptase, protease, and integrase. The reaction mechanisms of these enzymes have been studied using the QM-MM approach. Other examples are G-protein-coupled receptors, 5-HT_4 receptors, design and evaluation of a novel class of FKBP12 ligands, and novel inhibitors of human DHFR.

Table 10.1: Accuracy of different quantum mechanics methods

	Accuracy	*Maximum atoms*
Semiempirical	Low	2,000
Hartree–Fock and density functional	Medium	500
Perturbation and variation methods	High	50
Coupled cluster	Very high	20

11

Energy Minimization and Conformational Analysis

ENERGY MINIMIZATION METHODS

Energy minimization methods for knowing the stable conformers of a molecule are important because it allows us to understand properties and behaviour based upon structural considerations. When a molecule is built in a computational chemistry software package, the initial geometry does not necessarily correspond to one of the stable conformers. Therefore, energy minimization is usually carried out to determine a stable conformer; this same process is commonly referred to as geometry optimization.

Energy minimization is a numerical procedure for finding a minimum on the potential energy surface starting from a higher energy initial structure, labelled "1" as illustrated in Fig. 11.1. During energy minimization, the geometry is changed in a stepwise fashion so that the energy of the molecule is reduced, from steps 2 to 3 to 4 as shown in Fig. 11.1. After a number of steps, a local or global minimum on the potential energy surface is reached.

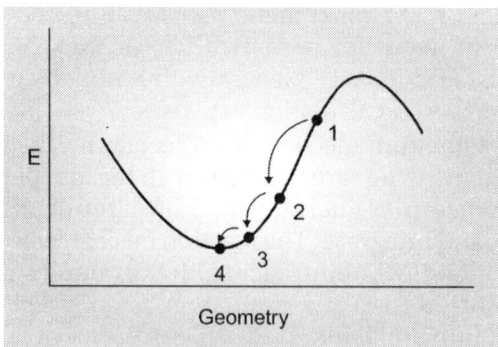

Fig. 11.1: The process of energy minimization changes the geometry of the molecule in a stepwise fashion until a minimum is reached

Most energy minimization methods proceed by determining the energy and the slope of the function at point 1. If the slope is positive, it is an indication that the coordinate is too large (as for point 1). If the slope is negative, then the coordinate is too small. The numerical minimization technique then adjusts the coordinate; if the slope is positive, the value of the coordinate is reduced as shown by point 2. The energy and the slope are again calculated for point 2. If the slope is zero, a minimum has been reached. If the slope is still positive, then the coordinate is reduced further, as shown for point 3, until a minimum is obtained.

There are numerous methods for actually varying the geometry to find the minimum; only a few will be discussed here. Many of the methods used to find a minimum on the potential energy surface of a molecule use an iterative formula and proceed in a step-wise fashion. These are all based on formulas of the type:

$$x_{new} = x_{old} + \text{correction} \tag{11.1}$$

In Eq. (11.1), x_{new} refers to the value of the geometry at the next step (for example, moving from step 1 to 2 in the figure), x_{old} refers to the geometry at the current step, and correction is some adjustment made to the geometry. In all these methods, a numerical test is applied to the new geometry (x_{new}) to decide if a minimum is reached. For example, the slope may be tested to see if it is zero within some numerical tolerance. If the criterion is not met, then the formula is applied again to make another change in the geometry.

Energy Minimization Methods

Energy minimization is used synonymously with geometry optimization categorised as:

- Derivative-based optimization algorithms that use derivatives of the energy function
- Nonderivative-based optimization algorithms that do not use derivatives of the energy function

Derivative Based Methods

- **First derivative methods**
  a. Steepest gradient
  b. Conjugate gradient method
- **Second derivative methods**
  Newton-Raphson method

Nonderivative Based Methods

- Simplex method
- Sequential univariate method

Steepest Descent Method

Rather than requiring the calculation of numerous second derivatives, the steepest descent method relies on an approximation. In this method, the second derivative is assumed to be a constant. Therefore, Eq. (11.1) to update the geometry becomes

$$x_{new} = x_{old} - \gamma \, E'(x_{old}) \tag{11.2}$$

where γ is a constant. In this method, the gradients at each point still must be calculated, but by not requiring second derivatives to be calculated, the method is much faster per step than the Newton–Raphson method. However, because of the approximation, it is not as efficient and so more steps are generally required to find the minimum.

The method is named *steepest descent* because the direction in which the geometry is first minimized is in the direction in which the gradient is largest (i.e. steepest) at the initial point. Once a minimum in the first direction is reached, a second minimization is carried out starting from that point and moving in the steepest remaining direction. This process continues until a minimum has been reached in all directions to within a sufficient tolerance. Such a process is illustrated for a system with two geometrical coordinates in Fig. 11.2.

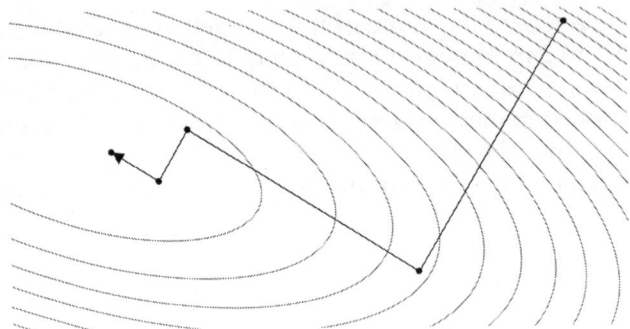

Fig.11.2: Illustration of the steepest descent method for a system with two geometrical coordinates

Conjugate Gradient Method

In this method, the first portion of the search takes place in the direction of the largest gradient, just as in the steepest descent method. However, to avoid some of the oscillating back and forth that often plagues the steepest descent method as it moves toward the minimum, the conjugate gradient method mixes in a little of the previous direction in the next search (Fig. 11.3). This allows the method to move rapidly to the minimum. The equations for the conjugate gradient method in two or more dimensions are more complex than those of the other two methods, so they will not be given here.

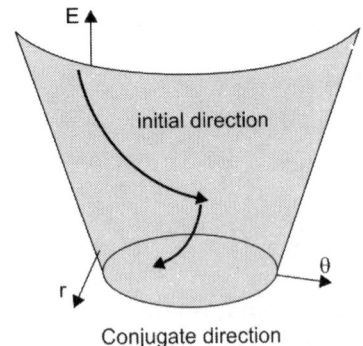

Fig. 11.3: Conjugate gradient method

Newton-Raphson Method

The Newton–Raphson method is the most computationally expensive per step of all the methods utilized to perform energy minimization. It is based on a Taylor series expansion of the potential energy surface at the current geometry.

The equation for updating the geometry

$$x_{new} = x_{old} - \frac{E'(X\,old)}{E''(X\,old)} \tag{11.3}$$

Notice that the correction term depends on both the first derivative (also called the slope or gradient) of the potential energy surface at the current geometry and also on the second derivative (otherwise known as the curvature). It is the necessity of calculating these derivatives at each step that makes the method very expensive per step, especially for a multidimensional potential energy surface where there are many directions in which to calculate the gradients and curvatures. However, the Newton–Raphson method usually requires the fewest steps to reach the minimum.

Simplex Method

Simplex is a geometrical figure with M+1 interconnected vertices, where M is the dimensionality of the energy function (Fig. 11.4), it does not rely on the calculation of the gradients at all. As a result, it is the least expensive in CPU time per step. However, it also often requires the more steps.

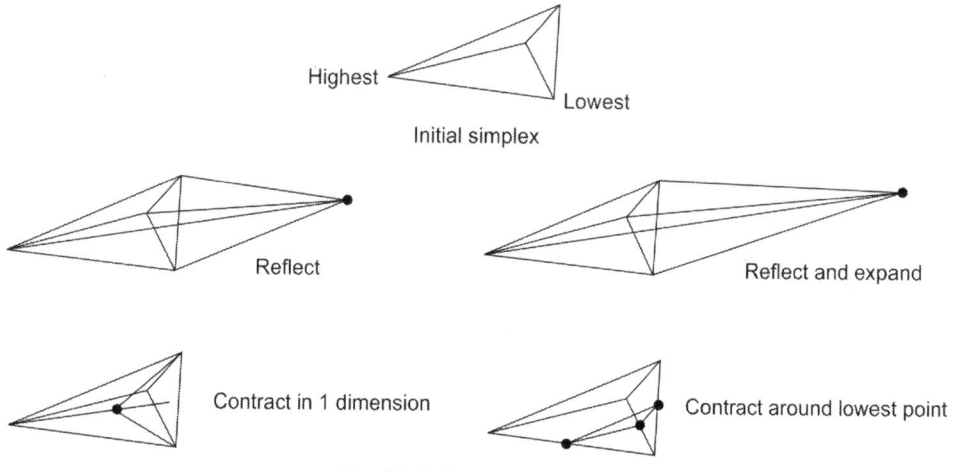

Fig. 11.4: Simplex method

To implement the simplex algorithm it is first necessary to generate the vertices of the initial simplex. The initial configuration of the system corresponds to just one of these vertices. The remaining points can be obtained by adding a constant increment to each coordinate in turn. The energy of the system is calculated at the new point, giving the function value for the relevant vertex. The point with the highest energy of the three is noted. Then, this point is reflected through the line segment connected the other two (to move away from the region of high energy). If the energy of point A is the highest out of the three points A, B and C, then A is reflected through line segment BC to produce point D (Fig. 11.5). In the next step, the two original lowest energy points (B and C) along with the new point D are analyzed. The highest energy point of these is selected, and that point is reflected through the line segment connecting the other two. The process continues until a minimum is located.

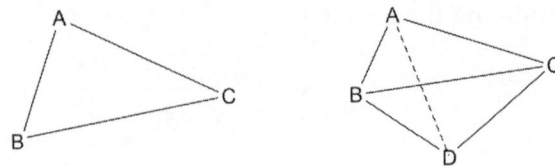

Fig. 11.5: Energy calculation of a system using simplex method

The Sequential Univariate Method

It is a nonderivative method that is considered more appropriate as it systematically cycles through the coordinates in turn. For each coordinate, two new structures are generated by changing the current coordinate. The energies of these two structures are calculated. A parabola is then fitted through the 3 points corresponding to the two distorted structures and the original structure. The minimum point in this quadratic function is determined and the coordinate is then changed to the position of the minimum.

An Example of the use of Energy Minimization Methods–CPU Times

As an example of these various energy minimization methods, the geometry of lactic acid was optimized using the Newton–Raphson, Steepest Descent, and Conjugate Gradient methods. Lactic acid is a relatively small organic molecule shown in Fig. 11.6.

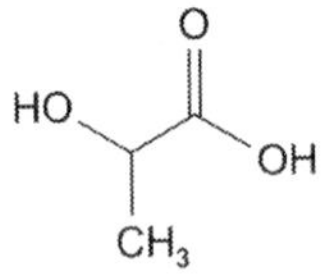

Fig. 11.6: Lactic acid

The results of the energy minimizations are summarized in Table 11.1. Each minimization started from the same initial geometry of lactic acid and used the same force field (MM3).

Table 11.1: Energy minimization of lactic acid using the MM3 force field			
Method	*No. of steps*	*Total CPU time (sec)*	*CPU time/step*
Newton–Raphson	15	14.8	0.99
Conjugate Gradient	72	15.8	0.22
Steepest Descent	500	41.0	0.08

From Table 1.1, it is clear that the Newton–Raphson method required the fewest number of steps to reach the minimum, while the Steepest Descent method required by far the largest number of steps. On the other hand, the Steepest Descent method required the smallest amount of CPU time per step, so even though it required 8-30 times more steps than the other methods, it only required about 2.7 fold more CPU time.

For larger molecules, the expense of the Newton–Raphson method becomes even more pronounced, leading to a much higher CPU time per step than for the other methods. Even though each step takes the smallest amount of CPU time of the three methods, the Steepest Descent method requires many more steps to find a minimum, so it is very inefficient. Therefore, the most commonly used method for energy minimization of large molecules is usually some form of the Conjugate Gradient method.

Applications

The energy minimization methods are used for:
- Comparison of structures/properties
- Template forcing
- Systematic mapping of E space
- Binding energies evaluation
- Docking
- Harmonic analysis
- Comparing/fitting force fields.

Conformational Analysis

The most significant concerns in medicinal chemistry and pharmaceutical research are structure elucidation, conformational analysis, physicochemical characterization and biological activity determination. The determination of molecular structure is necessary as the structure of the molecule predicts the physical, chemical, and biological properties of the molecule.

Conformational search methods find applications in the design of targeted chemical hosts and drug discovery. Conformations are different 3D spatial arrangements of the atoms in a molecule. They are interconvertible by free rotation of single bonds.

The major objective of conformational analysis is to gain insight on conformational characteristic of flexible biomolecules and drugs but to also identify the relation between the role of conformational flexibility and their activity. Therefore, it plays a significant role in computer-aided design as well. The significance of conformational analysis not just extends to computational docking and screening but also for lead optimization.

Conformational analysis: DHR Barton is considered the most important contributor to modern conformational analysis. In 1950, he proved how a variety of substituents at the equatorial and axial positions influence the rate of reactivity of substituted cyclohexanes. Identification of all possible minimum-energy structures (conformations) of a molecule is the main objective of conformational analysis.

It is a computational method in which commands are used such that the molecule assumes a conformation similar to the rigid template molecule. Conformational analysis is a difficult issue because even simple molecules may have a large number of conformational isomers. The usual strategy in conformational analysis is to use a search algorithm to generate a series of initial conformations.

Each of these conformations then subjected to energy minimization in order to derive the associated minimum energy structure.

Global minimum-energy conformation is the conformation with the lowest energy. It is not necessary that the global energy minimum conformation is the bioactive conformation of the drug. Most drugs behave like flexible molecules by means of distortions and rotations about rotatable bonds hence, adopt large number of conformations. Conformation analysis of pharmacophore becomes the most essential task in drug discovery.

Pharmacophore is a collection of steric and electronic features that are crucial to ensure optimal communication between the specific biological targets (Receptor/Enzyme) so as to give a biological response. The most difficult task in 3D pharmacophore recognition is the identification of the receptor bound/bioactive conformation. This can be done by studies of the spatial arrangement of the bioactive conformer so as to define the 3D pharmacophore. This conformation could be the local minimum, global minimum or any transition state between the local minima as shown in Fig. 11.7. Although it is common practice to assume that global minimum is the bioactive conformation.

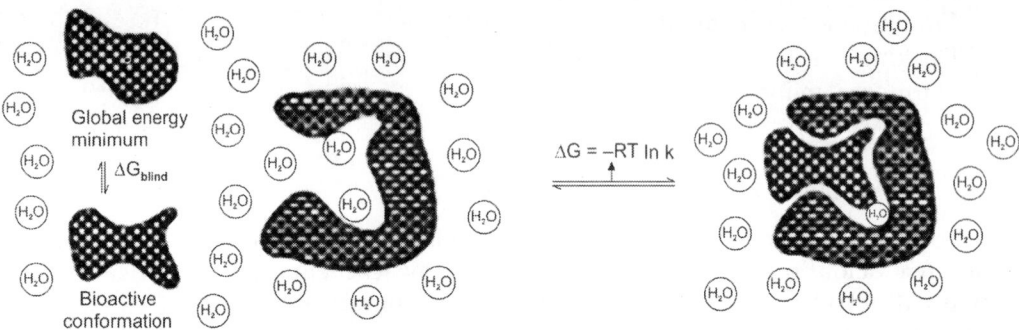

Fig. 11.7: The equilibrium characterizing the receptor–ligand complex interaction

To determine the information about conformations, different instrumental techniques are used like

- X-ray diffraction
- Electron diffraction
- Raman spectroscopy
- Ultraviolet spectroscopy
- Infra red spectroscopy
- NMR spectroscopy
- Microwave spectroscopy
- Photoelectron spectroscopy
- Supersonic molecular jet spectroscopy
- Optical rotatory dispersion and CD measurements
- Molecular mechanics

Conformation Search Methods

To get the best conformations, various types of search methods are available and discussed below:

- Conformational sampling
- Systematic search method
- Random searches

- Metropolis Monte Carlo methods
- Genetic algorithm and evolutionary algorithm
- Model building methods
- Molecular dynamics
- Distance geometry
- Neural networks
- Conformation optimization
- Conformational analysis

Conformational sampling: Conformation sampling is a procedure used to create a collection of molecular conformations that will later be analyzed. Ideally, all locally stable conformations of the molecule should be reported for in order for the conformational analysis to be complete. As the size of the molecule increases, the number of locally stable conformations increases so fast that the task of full enumeration becomes formidable. The basic prerequisite is that the resulting conformational sample "ensemble" will be representative of the system as a whole.

Systematic search method: In this method, there is systemic generation of conformations and thus exploration of the conformational space through assigning of discrete values to torsion angles of rotatable bonds of the drug which results in regular and predictable alterations of the structure. The values are limited to a set of predetermined values. In systematic search, exploration of the energy surface of the molecule is carried out in a predictable pattern. It is used where it's not possible to predict the order in which conformations will be generated by random methods.

Grid search is the simplest type of systematic search algorithm in which conformations corresponding to all possible combinations of torsion angle values are generated. Series of conformations are generated by systematic rotation of torsion angles around the rotatable single bonds between angles of $0°$ and $360°$. For example, if a molecule has two variable torsion angles such that the first torsion angle can adopt the values $60°$, $180°$ and $60°$ and the second torsion angle may adopt values $0°$ and $180°$. Six conformations will be generated by the grid search (i.e. $60°$, $0°$; $60°$, $180°$; $180°$, $0°$; $180°$, $180°$; $60°$, $0°$; $60°$; $180°$)[6]. The number of conformations is given by; S^N, where N is the number of free rotation angles, S is the number of discrete values for each rotation angle. $S = 360/\varphi i$; φi being the dihedral increment of angle i. Due to the exponential increase in number of conformations increases due to the number of bonds that have free rotation lead to combinatorial complexity, which is most crucial drawback involved in a systematic search. Building molecules from aggregates or by the use of distance constraint equations are some methods that help in resolving the combinatorial explosion.

Random searches: Random search is the exact opposite of systematic search. It can move from one region of the conformational space to a completely unconnected new region in a single step. Random search methods can study conformational spaces either changing the atomic cartesian coordinates or torsion angles of rotable bonds. A number of random conformational search methods have been devised. They all generally involve a repetitive procedure in which an initial structure is selected, randomly modified and minimized. At each step random change is made to the current conformer found and structure is refined using energy minimization. The conformation generated is added to the list of structures found. This conformation is starting point for next step and the sequence is repeated. Since there is no natural end point; the process continues until either a predefined number of iterations have been attempted and/or until no new conformations are generated.

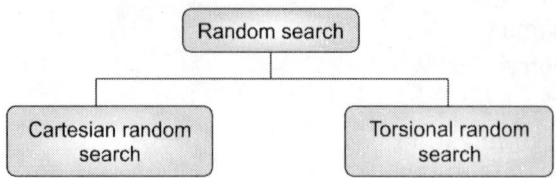

Table 11.2: Differences between Cartesian random search and torsional random search

S. No.	Cartesian random search	Torsional random search
1.	Addition of random amount to x, y and z coordinates of all atoms in a molecule occurs.	Random change to torsion angles of rotable bonds are made such that bond lengths and bond angles are kept fixed.
2.	Implementation is simple but relies deeply on energy minimization as structures generated can be disoriented or have extremely high energy.	Special procedures are needed to change torsional angles in molecules containing rings as ring constraints must be fulfilled in each ring.

Monte Carlo method: Monte Carlo method is one of the important methods as it was the technique used to execute the first computer simulation of a molecular system. The method is based on statistical mechanics. Monte Carlo minimum method (MCMM) is a single starting geometry used repeatedly to accumulate its progeny. An important feature of this method is that the Monte Carlo scheme can study, sample and calculate energy of all the states. The Boltzmann weight contribution to the average can also be calculated. In simple stochastic search, from a given starting structure random alterations are made and internal energy of resulting structure is calculated and energy minimization is undertaken. The new conformer produces is saved if the energy or the difference in energies between the new and the best conformer is less than the threshold optimum energy (ΔE) value.

$$\Delta E < \Delta E_{MIN}$$
$$\Delta E - E_{MIN}, \Delta E$$

The search is automatically concluded after a user defined number of unproductive attempts. The termination number is set at about a few hundred. The Monte–Carlo method has been successfully used to find minimum energy conformations for cycloalkanes using specific constraint conditions, but cannot generally be extended to unrestricted systems. Monte–Carlo method is appropriate for large molecules with complex interconversion pathway.

Systematic unbounded minimum method (SUMM): It is a variant of the Monte Carlo method. The SUMM approach of Goodman and Still suggests a new internal coordinate transversal of conformational space. Low resolution (120° torsion angle space) generates torsionally remote conformers early on in the search method. It appears to be more efficient at finding low energy conformations for medium and large ring molecules.

Random incremental pulse search (RIPS): In this method, starting with input geometry, random changes (±1 Å) is preformed on the coordinates of each atom or a subset of atoms and the perturbed geometry is then subjected to minimization to find new conformers.

Metropolis Monte Carlo method: The approach amplifies the chances of finding the global minimum. It involves number of sequences where the Monte Carlo Algorithm is run at different temperatures. The first phase runs at temperature T_1 and an assortment of conformations are generated. The most stable conformation is used as starting origin for next phase where temperature is set at lower temperature. The process is repeated until the probability equation becomes selective towards which structure is accepted. Thus a small part of the conformation space is meticulously investigated. Similar to stochastic method it introduces probability parameter to accept new conformers. The *Boltzmann factor* is calculated using the formula

$$P = \exp^{-\Delta E / K_b T} \tag{11.4}$$

where P is the, probability criteria, ΔE Energy factor, K_b is the Boltzmann constant, and T is similar to temperature in Boltzmann is the law and is termed *temperature* by analogy.

The acceptance test is performed by choosing a random number (between 0 and 1) and evaluating it against the probability factor ($\exp^{-\Delta E / K_b T}$). If the random number is lower, the change is accepted and new conformation is yielded which can be used as the new starting point. Also If the Boltzmann factor is larger than a random number between zero and one then the new structure is selected. If not then the previous structure is retained.

Genetic algorithm: Genetic algorithms are a class of optimization methods that are based on various computational models of Darwinian evolution. A genetic algorithm is a large-scale optimization algorithm mimicking a biological evolution in a randomly generated population. A number of conformations are available from this population. The adaptation is calculated, and a new population is created in accordance to operators (crossover, and mutation). The process is repeated until it converges to a minimum energy structure. Selection of the initial population of conformers analogous to parent is carried out with a statistical bias such that only stable conformations are selected. The chromosome represented by torsional angles or any other parameter may alter due to crossover or mutation resulting in new and diversified conformers. The process may be repeated for as long as it is practically possible. Stable configurations may be formed early and can be lost due to crossover or mutation. To prevent this most programs have an elitist strategy to carry forward the most stable conformations.

Model building approaches: The assumptions of the model building approach are: (a) Each of the fragments must be conformationally independent of the other fragments of the molecule (b) Each fragment conformations stored must cover range of structures that are observed in the completely built molecule.

In this model, construction of conformation of the molecule is done by fusion of three dimensional structures of molecular fragments. It is expected to be more effective than normal systematic search as the number of combinations of fragment conformations is less than that of the combination of torsional angles or Cartesian coordinates. The program must decide which fragments are required to construct the molecule. This is accomplished by utilizing the sub culture search algorithm, which determines whether each of fragments that program knows about is present and how they match onto the atoms in the molecule.

Molecular dynamics: Molecular dynamics is a conformational space search procedure in which the atoms of molecule are given an initial velocity and are then allowed to evolve in time according to the laws of Newtonian mechanics. In this method, generation of successive configurations is carried out by incorporation of Newton's law of motion for the atoms in the system, to provide a *trajectory* that defines how the positions and velocities of the particles of the system vary with time. Molecular dynamics is a computer program that treats the atoms within the molecules as moving spheres. After 10^{-15} sec of movement, determination of the position and velocity of each atom in structure is used for the estimation of the forces by utilizing the values of bond lengths, bond angles, torsional terms and non-bonded interactions. The calculation of potential energy of each atom and Newton's Law of Motion helps in the computation of acceleration and direction of each atom. Generation of different conformations is carried out by program by "Heating" of molecule which implies that the molecule undergoes bond stretching and bond rotation as if it was being heated. The process can be repeated automatically to give any number of practical structures. Molecular Dynamics thus provides not only information about the conformation system but also the way in which the conformation changes with time. Twist boat conformation of cyclo hexane is not the most stable form but molecular dynamic program predicts a more stable chair form .

Distance geometry: Distance geometry uses the interatomic distances and various mathematical procedures to generate structures of conformations for energy minimization. In this method, a set of distance constraints is transformed into a set of Cartesian coordinates. The limitation is that it is not possible to randomly assign interatomic distance values in a molecule and low energy conformations are formed as a result of this feature The distances are calculated according to bond angles, and torsion angles for free and rigid angles, and any other known constraints on the system. These distances are taken into a matrix and lower and upper bounds are represented. Derivation of a conformation by Distance geometry occurs in four stages.

Stage 1: Matrix containing the maximum and minimum values permitted to each interatomic distance in the molecule is calculated.

Stage 2: Each interatomic distance is arbitrarily assigned values between the upper and lower bounds.

Stage 3: Distance Matrix is transformed into trial set of artesian coordinates.

Stage 4: Refinement of structure and generation of conformation is the last stage.

Refinement of structure is carried out in accordance to simple trigonometric restrictions. The distance between A and C can be no greater than the sum of maximum values of distances between AB and BC.

$$U_{AC} > U_{AB} + U_{BC}$$

Minimum value of AC distance can be no less than the difference between the lower bound on AB and the upper bound on BC:

$$L_{AC} < L_{AB} - U_{BC}$$

The distance matrix is subjected to a process called embedding, In which the distance space is representation of conformation is converted to a set of atomic Cartesian coordinates. This generates the conformation. The method is applicable to conformational search on small or medium size molecules.

Neural networks: Artificial neural networks are based on the concepts that were motivated by the theories of the cell network of the human brain. Neural networks are designed to mimic the information processing and knowledge acquisition of the human brain. They have basic segments called artificial neurons that perform identical tasks. They are generally applied to nonlinear problems and pattern recognition studies. In conformational analysis, neural networks have been used to predict the maximum and minimum distances between pairs of heteroatoms. It is used in studies related to protein folding, secondary structure, location of disulfide bridges and surface accessible of each residue.

Conformational optimization: The various sampling procedures result in a number of transient conformations. During energy minimization of these structures is to bring these conformations to the minima before analysis is performed. Minimization methods are used as a tool in model building, preparation of the initial structure for molecular dynamics and groundwork of structures for normal mode analysis.

Stimulated annealing is used in optimizing the problems where minimization of objective function can be carried out without being caught in local minima. It is designed for finding the global minimum and samples low energy conformations more sharply. It is derived by analogy with the process of crystallization; slow cooling produces stable crystalline forms corresponding to global minimum, whereas rapid freezing may lead to the formation of metastable form corresponding to local minimum. Stimulated annealing is monitored by a cooling schedule and the process is broken up into a number of cycles, each at constant temperature and composed of large number of individual levels corresponding to stochastic search with Metropolis criterion. Each level is believed to be producing Boltzmann distribution.

The temperature is lowered and process is repeated. Alternatively it can be said that heating up the system provides the molecule the energy facilitating it to leap out of its initial local minimum. The gradual cooling that is consequently applied decreases the amplitude of these vibrations and conveys the particulars of the energy surface back into focus and causes the system to gradually settle down to a lower energy minimum. Due to progressive decrease in temperature explorations of conformations of decreasing cost can analyze smaller and smaller regions of conformational space such that system falls into global minimum.

Conformational analysis: The analysis of the conformational collection that was sampled and optimized is essential so as to ascertain the conformational properties of the molecule that is being studied. This helps to underline the global properties and to exemplify features of overall flexibility and to recognize common inclination in the conformation set. Alternatively, it may be used to identify a smaller subset of characteristic low energy conformations, which may be used to direct future drug development efforts.

Some methods of conformational analysis are given below:

a. Similarity measures: A similarity measure is essential for quantitative comparison of one structure with another and it must be defined before the analysis. Structural similarity is calculated by a root-mean-square distance (RMSD) between two conformations. In Cartesian coordinates the RMS distance *dij* between conformation *i* and conformation *j* of a given molecule is defined as the minimum of the functional

$$d_{ij} = \left[\frac{1}{N} \sum_{i=j}^{N} \left| r_k^{(i)} - r_k^{(j)} \right|^2 \right]^{1/2} \tag{11.5}$$

where, N is the number of atoms in the summation, k is an index over these atoms, $r_k^{(i)}$, $r_k^{(j)}$ are the Cartesian coordinates of atom k in conformations i and j.

b. Cluster analysis: Cluster analysis is a regular investigative technique used to group conformations. In this method structural similarity are highlighted and are defined by the distance measure being used within a conformational sample. The initial conformation selected is generally of low energy and all conformations that are contained by a given cutoff distance from this structure are grouped together to form first cluster. The ungrouped conformations are selected and new cluster is formed. The procedure is repeated until all conformations are assigned into clusters. In many conformational studies, cluster analysis is used as a way to focus future effort on a small set of characteristic conformations.

One conformation, typically the lowest energy one, is picked from each of the highly populated conformational clusters. The resulting small number of distinctly different conformations are then used as starting points for further computational analysis (such as free energy simulations) or as a basis for generating a pharmacological hypothesis used for directing future drug development.

Applications

- Used in the refinement of X-ray and NMR data to determine the three dimensional structures of large biological molecules such as protein, automated docking of substrates to proteins and thus in protein engineering.
- The generation of Quantitative Structure–Activity Relationships (QSAR) models.
- Receptor modeling, particularly regarding the binding of small ligand molecules to sites of proteins or macromolecules.
- Use of conformational restriction in drug design: The constrained systematic search procedure was used in the discovery of 3D pharmacophores for the inhibition of Angiotensin Converting Enzyme (ACE), an enzyme involved in the regulation of blood pressure.
- Design and analysis of compound library.

Appendices

Appendix 1: Computer-aided techniques used in drug design and discovery	
Technique	*Roles in drug design and discovery*
Docking	Predict binding mode and approximate binding energy of a compound to a target
Structure-based virtual screening	Identify active compounds for a specific target from a chemical library based on docking techniques
Pharmacophore modeling	Perceive and provide description of molecular features necessary for molecular recognition of a ligand by a biological macromolecule
Ligand-based virtual screening	Identify active compounds for a specific target from a chemical library based on pharmacophore modeling techniques
Homology modeling	Build a 3D structure for structure-based drug design for a target for which no crystal structure is available, based on related protein 3D structures
Molecular dynamics	Molecular mechanics-based simulation to understand the dynamic behavior of proteins or other biological macromolecules, to analyze the flexibility of the drug target for structure-based drug design and/or to calculate the binding affinity of a compound to a target
2D quantitative structure–activity relationship	Finding a model that can be used to predict some property from the molecular structure of a compound
3D quantitative structure–activity relationship	Technique used to quantitatively predict the interaction between a molecule and the active site of a target; 3D conformation-derived information is utilized in this technique
Quantum mechanics	An electron-orbital-based approach based on first principles to optimize structures of ligands and even protein–ligand complexes, improve the accuracy of docking and calculate, for example, free-binding energy
Absorption, distribution, metabolism, elimination, and toxicity prediction	Prediction of absorption, distribution, metabolism, elimination and toxicity of chemical substances in the human body to avoid costly later-stage failures in drug development

Appendix 2: Commercial software packages for drug design		
Name	*Owned and distributed by*	*Modules*
Discovery Studio	Accelrys Inc.	• Biopolymer: building and editing macromolecular structures • Catalyst: pharmacophore generation • CHARMM: molecular dynamics • LigandFit: shape-based docking • LibDock: feature-based docking • LUDI: *de novo* design • Modeller: homology modeling • Quantitative structure–activity relationship (QSAR): QSAR modeling • TOPKAT: ADME/T prediction • VAMP: semiempirical QM program • ZDOCK and RDOCK: protein–protein docking
ICM	Molsoft LLC	• ICM Browser Pro: molecular graphics and visualization • ICM Homology: homology modeling • ICM Pro: small-molecule docking, protein–protein docking, protein structure prediction • ICM Chemist: display and manipulation of chemical datasets, chemical searching, pharmacophore searching, display chemical data, QSAR prediction • ICM VLS: virtual screening
LeadIT	BioSolveIT GmbH	• FlexX: ligand docking • FlexX-Pharm: pharmacophore type constraint docking • FlexX-Ensemble: flexible receptor docking • FlexS: 3D alignment of small molecules • FTrees: similarity search • CoLibri: creation, management and manipulation of ligand fragments • ReCore: novel scaffold hopping in the binding site • FlexNovo: fragment-based design of compounds
MOE	Chemical Computing Group	• Structure-based design: scaffold replacement; ligand-receptor docking; multifragment search; LigX: ligand optimization in pocket • Pharmacophore discovery • Chemoinformatics and (high-throughput screening) QSAR • Protein and antibody modeling: homology modeling and macromolecular simulation • Molecular modeling and simulations: conformation generation, analysis, and clustering
OpenEye[†]	OpenEye Scientific Software Inc.	• BROOD: bioisosteric replacements search • EON: electrostatics comparison • FILTER: molecular filtering and selection application • FRED: ligand docking and scoring • OMEGA: generation of 3D conformer ensembles • QUACPAC: tautomer/protomer enumeration • ROCS: shape (and chemistry) similar search

(Contd.)

Appendix 2: Commercial software packages for drug design		
Name	*Owned and distributed by*	*Modules*
		• SZYBKI: structure optimization *in situ* with MMFF94 • VIDA: graphical interface for visualization
Schrödinger	Schrödinger Inc.	• Canvas: chemoinformatics • CombiGlide: combinatorial technology • ConfGen: bioactive conformation generation • Core Hopping: novel scaffolds discovery • Desmond: molecular dynamics • Epik: fast pK_a and tautomer prediction • Glide: docking and scoring • Impact: molecular mechanics and dynamics • Jaguar: quantum mechanics • Konstanz Information Miner extensions: workflow/pipelining • Liaison: relative binding affinity prediction • LigPrep: 3D structure generation • MacroModel: a general purpose, force field-based molecular modeling program • MOPAC: semiempirical quantum chemistry • MCPRO+: Monte Carlo simulations • Phase: pharmacophore modeling • Prime: homology modeling • PrimeX: protein crystal structure refinement • QikProp: ADME/T prediction • QSite: quantum mechanics/molecular mechanics • SiteMap: protein binding site identification and analysis • Strike: QSAR, statistical modelling
SYBYL	Tripos Inc.	• Biopolymer: predict and build macromolecular 3D structure • CombiLibMaker: generate virtual combinatorial libraries • Concord: 3D structure generation • Confort: conformers generation • DISCOtech: pharmacophore model building • Distill: determine and visualize structure–activity relationships • DiverseSolutions: design, compare, or select compound libraries • GALAHAD: pharmacophoric perception and molecular alignments • GASP: pharmacophore hypotheses building • Legion: construct virtual combinatorial libraries • RACHEL: optimization of lead compounds • Selector: characterize and sample compound libraries • Surflex-Dock: docking and virtual screening • Tuplets: pharmacophore-based virtual screening without a 3D model • UNITY: 3D database searching

Name	Developed by	Incorporated into software package	Free for academia	Drug-design applications
AutoDock	Scripps Research Institute[†]	–	Yes	Aldose reductase inhibitors Rac1 Inhibitors Trypanothione reductase inhibitors
DOCK	University of California, San Francisco[‡]	–	Yes	STAT3 dimerization inhibitors Death-associated protein kinase inhibitors Inhibitors of osteoclast formation and bone resorption
FlexX	BioSolveIT GmbH	LeadIT	No	Inhibitors of penicillin binding protein Inhibitors of ATP-phosphoribosyl transferase Human histamine H4 receptor ligands
FRED	OpenEye Scientific Software	Open Eye	Yes	Proteasome inhibitors Heat-shock protein 90 inhibitors
Glide	Schrödinger, Inc.	Schrödinger	No	Inhibitors of dengue virus methyltransferase FGFR1 kinase inhibitors HIV-1 integrase inhibitors
GOLD	Cambridge Crystallographic Data Centre	-	No	Topoisomerase I inhibitors MNK1 inhibitors Met tyrosine kinase inhibitors
ICM	Molsoft LLC.	Molsoft	No	TNF-á inhibitors Aryl hydrocarbon receptor ligands GTP competitive inhibitors
Surflex-Dock	Tripos Inc.	SYBYL	No	Glycogen synthase kinase inhibitors Proteasome inhibitors HIV-1 reverse transcriptase inhibitors

Appendix 3: The most used docking programs in structure-based drug design

Appendix 4: Commonly used pharmacophore modeling programs				
Name	*Developed by*	*Incorporated into software package*	*Methods*	*Drug design applications*
Catalyst	Accelrys Inc.	Discovery Studio	Ligand based, includes the two methods HipHop and HypoGen for pharmacophore perception Produces conformers using pre-enumerating method by the Poling algorithm Uses feature-based method to align molecules	Acetylcholinesterase inhibitors $\sigma 1$ receptor ligands Tubulin inhibitors
DISCO tech	Tripos Inc.	SYBYL	Ligand based Produces conformers using pre-enumerating method by Concord and Confort Uses Bron–Kerbosh clique-detection algorithm to align molecules	Glycogen synthase kinase inhibitors SGLT2 inhibitors Ligands of AT2
Ligand Scout	Inte:Ligand[†]		Structure based Pharmacophoric feature points-based pattern-matching alignment algorithm	11 β-HSD1 inhibitors Pim1 inhibitors HIV-1 transcriptase inhibitors
MOE	Chemical Computing Group	MOE	Ligand based Produces conformers using pre-enumerating method by various methods ranging from molecular dynamics to stochastic methods and systematic search Uses property-based algorithm to align molecules	Antitubercular agentsReversal agentsAntimalarial agents
PHASE	Schrödinger, Inc.	Schrödinger	Ligand based Produces conformers using pre-enumerating method by ConfGen Uses feature-based algorithm to align molecules	Inhibitors of dengue virus methyl-transferase Selective MDR1 agents γ-aminobutyric acid G1 receptor $\rho 1$ antagonists

Appendix 5: Databases of interest for drug discovery

Database	Publisher	License type
Open National Cancer Institute Database	National Cancer Institute	Publicly available
PubChem	National Center for Biotechnology Information	Publicly available
BindingDB	University of Maryland, USA	Publicly available
Relibase	Cambridge Crystallographic Data Centre	Freely accessible for academia, commercial version available
ChEMBLdb	European Bioinformatics Institute, Hinxton, UK	Publicly available
ChemSpider	Royal Society of Chemistry, UK	Publicly available
Human Metabolome Database	University of Alberta, Canada	Publicly available
World Drug Index	Thomson Reuters	Commercial

Appendix 6: Major molecular dynamics programs used in drug design

Name	Developed by	Free for academia	Drug design applications
Amber	University of California, San Francisco, USA[†]	No	Human acetylcholinesterase inhibitors HIV-1 reverse transcriptase inhibitors
CHARMM	Harvard University, USA[‡]	No	Glucose binding to insulin Flaviviral protease inhibitors
Desmond	D. E. Shaw Research[§]	Yes	
GROMACS	University of Groningen, The Netherlands[¶]	Yes	Antiviral compounds for avian influenza neuraminidase
NAMD	University of Illinois, USA[#]	Yes	

Appendix 7: Quantum mechanics programs with frequent use in drug design		
Name	*Developed by*	*Free for academia*
Gamess	Iowa State University, USA	Yes
Gaussian	Gaussian Inc.	No
Ghemical	University of Kuopio, Finland	Yes
Jaguar	Schrödinger Inc.	No
MOPAC	Stewart Computational Chemistry	Yes
NWChem	Environmental Molecular Sciences Laboratory	Yes
SPARTAN	Wavefunction, Inc.	No

Appendix 8: Available ADME/T prediction programs			
Program	*Developed by*	*Free for academia*	*Prediction spectrum*
ADMET Predictor	Simulations Plus, Inc.	No[†]	ADME/T
StarDrop	Optibrium, Ltd	No	ADME/T
ADME Suite Tox Suite	Advanced Chemistry Development, Inc.	No	ADME Toxicity
ADMEWORKS Predictor	Fujitsu FQS	No	ADME/T
Sarchitect	Strand Life Sciences	No	ADME/T
QikProp	Schrödinger, Inc.	No	ADME/T
TOPKAT	Accelrys, Inc.	No	Toxicity
Leadscope	Leadscope, Inc.	No	Toxicity
Meteor Derek Nexus	Lhasa, Ltd	No	Metabolism Toxicity
PASS	Russian Academy of Medical Sciences	No	Toxicity
Hazard Expert Pro MetabolExpert ToxAlert MEXAlert RetroMex	CompuDrug, Ltd	No	Toxicity Metabolism Toxicity Metabolism Metabolism
METAPC CASETOX	Multicase, Inc.	No	Metabolism Toxicity
VolSurf+MetaSite	Molecular Discovery, Ltd.	No	ADME Metabolism
Bioclipse	Uppsala University, Sweden and European Bioinformatics Institute	Yes	Metabolism
MetaDrug	GeneGo, Inc.	No	Metabolism/Toxicity
TIMES	OASIS Lmc	No	Metabolism/Toxicity

Question Bank

Questions on drug discovery and stages of drug development
1. What is drug discovery?
2. What are the different stages involved in drug development?
3. Explain the various phases of clinical trials?
4. What is the Indian scenario in handling drugs?

Questions on lead discovery and drug design
5. What is drug design?
6. What are the rational approaches to lead discovery?
7. What is serendipitous drug discovery? Explain with suitable examples.
8. What are the methods involved in lead discovery?
9. What is lead optimisation?
10. Explain lead discovery based upon clinical observations.

Questions on Bioisosterism
11. What is bioisosterism?
12. Classify bioisosters.
13. Discuss the case studies involved in bioisosterism.
14. Explain the various replacements of bioisosters.
15. What are the applications of bioisosterism in drug discovery with examples?

Questions on QSAR: Part I
16. What do you mean by QSAR?
17. What are the different parameters/descriptors used in QSAR?
18. What is the Craig's plot?
19. What are the steric factors?
20. Explain Hansch equation.
21. What is Free Wilson Analysis?

Questions on QSAR: Part II
22. What are the objectives of QSAR?
23. What are the methodologies of QSAR?
24. What are the 3D QSAR approaches?
25. What is CoMFA? Explain in detail alongwith its applications and drawbacks.
26. What is CoMSIA? Give its applications.
27. Differentiate between QSAR and SAR.

Questions on molecular modeling
28. What is molecular modeling? Discuss its methods and applications in drug designing.
29. What is molecular docking? Give its applications.
30. Describe the various force fields used in molecular docking.
31. What are various molecular modeling techniques?

32. What is scoring? Describe its method and functions involved.
33. What is *de novo* drug design? Explain various steps involved in computer-based drug designing.

Questions on virtual screening

34. Define virtual screening.
35. What is druglikeness screening? Explain the methods involved to calculate the druglikeness.
36. What is Pharamcophore concept in CADD?
37. What is Pharmacophore mapping?
38. Explain the applications and the limitations of pharmacophore screening in drug design.

Questions on cheminformatics and bioinformatics

39. What is Bioinformatics?
40. Which are the main sub disciplines of bioinformatics?
41. What is cheminformatics?
42. What is chemical genomics?
43. Describe the applications of cheminformatics in pharma industry.
44. What is the main role of a bioinformatician in present biological research and development area?

Questions on database

45. Define term database.
46. Which types of databases are used in bioinformatics?
47. Explain molecular mechanics and quantum mechanics?
48. What is data mining?
49. Explain the ADME related properties?
50. Which types of issues or problems related to biochemical data are dealt with the bioinformatics?

Questions on energy minimisation and conformational analysis

51. What is the concept of energy minimisation?
52. Explain the various methods involved in energy minimisation.
53. What are the applications of energy minimisation in drug discovery?
54. What is conformational analysis?
55. What is global minimum energy determination?
56. Explain the various search methods involved in conformational analysis.
57. Write down the applications of conformational analysis in drug designing.

Questions on molecular mechanics and quantum mechanics

58. What is molecular mechanics?
59. Give the applications of molecular mechanics in drug designing.
60. What are the limitations of molecular mechanics?
61. Define quantum mechanics.
62. What are the applications of quantum mechanics?
63. What is Schrödinger's wave mechanics?
64. Differentiate between quantum mechanics and molecular mechanics.

Index